EMOTIONAL HEALTH
AND WELL-BEING

EMOTIONAL HEALTH
AND WELL-BEING

Practical Mind Science

Jan Alcoe
and
Emily Gajewski

MERCURY LEARNING AND INFORMATION

Dulles, Virginia | Boston, Massachusetts | New Delhi

Publisher: David Pallai
MERCURY LEARNING AND INFORMATION
22841 Quicksilver Drive
Dulles, VA 20166
info@merclearning.com
www.merclearning.com
1-800-758-3756

This book is printed on acid-free paper.

Jan Alcoe and Emily Gajewski. *Emotional Health and Well-Being.*
ISBN: 978-1-938549-22-9

The publisher recognizes and respects all marks used by companies,
manufacturers, and developers as a means to distinguish their products. All
brand names and product names mentioned in this book are trademarks or
service marks of their respective companies. Any omission or misuse (of any
kind) of service marks or trademarks, etc. is not an attempt to infringe on the
property of others.

Library of Congress Control Number: 2013944478

131415321

Printed in the United States of America

The sole remedy in the event of a claim of any kind is expressly limited
to replacement of the book and/or disc, and only at the discretion of the
Publisher. The use of "implied warranty" and certain "exclusions" vary
from state to state, and might not apply to the purchaser of this product(see
complete license and disclaimer on page ii).

Our titles are available for adoption, license, or bulk purchase by
associations, universities, corporations, etc.
For additional information, please contact the Customer Service Dept. at
1-800-758-3756 (toll free) or info@merclearning.com.

For our children, who teach us daily
about wise living and well-being

Contents

Acknowledgments

In recognition of the research into emotional well-being by the Human Givens Institute, UK, and the inspiration we have had from the teaching of Ivan Tyrrell and Joe Griffin (Human Givens Institute), Mark Tyrrell (Uncommon Knowledge), and Jill Wooton (Within Sight).

Introduction

Welcome to *Emotional Health and Well-being*. If you have selected this book, you may be looking for practical ways of improving your well-being. If you are a health and well-being practitioner or therapist, you may be helping your patients to improve theirs by encouraging them to practice some of the approaches it is based on. Emotional health and well-being are subjective states of "feeling good" which have physical, mental, emotional, and even spiritual dimensions. This book is designed to provide information and a variety of routes to recovering, sustaining, protecting, and enhancing well-being, depending on your interests, needs, and motivations.

As you dip into this question and answer guide, you will be learning about and using a wide range of ideas and techniques from the broad field of contemporary psychology, including cognitive behavioral therapy, cognitive mindfulness, occupational therapy, clinical hypnotherapy, Human Givens therapy, positive psychology, compassion-focused therapy, and Neuro-linguistic programming (NLP) to improve your emotional health and well-being. All these approaches have evolved from research into our innate mental resources and the strong links between our thinking, emotions and behavior. This guide will steer you around the pitfalls of negative thinking, harmful emotions and stress-led behaviors which will impair your physical and mental well-being. You can then learn how to use your own mental resources in positive ways to meet your needs, whether to improve your physical health, boost your confidence or motivation, keep calm in the face of challenge, or reach peak performance.

The book includes many practical activities for you to try out, including short *"Try this"* ideas within the main text, and longer exercises on the accompanying CD-ROM. At the back of the book you will find key references and useful resources so you can find out more about subjects which interest you, together with a glossary of technical terms. These terms are highlighted in blue when mentioned in the text.

We have organized the questions and answers into categories of common challenges and needs which we may come across in our lives. Here is a summary of the main chapters:

Chapter 1: Laying the Foundations of Emotional Health and Well-being

The first chapter will help you to lay down some important foundation stones for well-being, based on the science of the mind. It introduces an evidence-based list of emotional needs which are essential to well-being and happiness. You can rate how well you are getting those needs met and begin to plan some positive changes. You will learn about the importance of "switching off" the body's **fight-or-flight response** when it is not needed, thus avoiding many stress-related health problems. You can try some effective techniques for deep relaxation based on **mindfulness** and visualization. You can begin to identify and connect with internal and external resources which you can draw on to support your well-being, particularly in challenging times. All these practices underpin the contents of this book. Learning to use them will enable you to harness the power of your mind to enhance well-being on many levels.

Chapter 2: Dealing with Stress, Anxiety, Panic, and Worry

The **fight-or-flight response** can be triggered by our fears, anxiety and worry and can sometimes lead us into a full-blown panic attack. This section will help you to avoid unnecessary stress in your life by concentrating on what you <u>can</u> change. You will learn how to evoke a sense of calm in stressful situations, and how to handle or avoid panic attacks to help you stay in control of your life. You can practice techniques for reducing the amount of time spent worrying and some emergency strategies for distracting away from fear, anxiety, and worry. Reducing your response to stress in these ways will enhance your well-being and put you back in control of your life. This chapter also covers more severe forms of anxiety and common psychological treatments.

Chapter 3: Controlling Negative Thinking and Avoiding Depression

How we think is closely linked to how we feel and how we then act in our lives. We can sometimes believe that we <u>are</u> our thoughts and this can lead us into a state of hopelessness and helplessness. Negative thinking can trigger the **fight-or-flight response** and is at the heart of depression. This chapter will help you to separate yourself from your thoughts, so that you can be objective about their content. You can learn about common errors of thinking so that you can guard against them. It is important to challenge negative thoughts and consciously change them, and there are several techniques included for doing just this. Finally, we cover the importance of understanding the symptoms and cycle of depression which can be triggered by constant, negative thinking, called **rumination.** Learning to avoid this pattern of thinking will help to ensure that you continue experiencing motivation and pleasure in life.

Chapter 4: Reducing Anger

Uncontrolled rage and anger are extremely destructive to our health, relationships, property, and community. Our daily lives can often include so little "down time" that stress levels have the ability to creep up and up to the point where we literally boil over. If you are someone with trauma or unresolved emotional difficulties from the past, you are also more likely to be at the mercy of uncontrolled anger. Whilst feeling angry at injustice or wrongdoing in the world can spur us forward to do something productive, uncontrolled outbursts of anger lead only downward, and at their worst can be life-threatening. This section explains what is going on in the brain when anger starts to rise and what we can do to prevent this happening. You can learn strategies to nip it in the bud so that you just don't get to boiling point, and how to review and change how you react in anger-provoking situations. This will help you to keep your rational mind in charge of your life so you can live your life how you would like to, more of the time.

Chapter 5: Improving Physical Health and Sleep

There is more and more research which demonstrates the interconnections between the brain, behavior, immunity, and health. For example, how we use our minds, including our thoughts, expectations and how we interpret life's events, can greatly impact upon our body's cellular activity and immunity and a whole host of physiological functions. This chapter will help you learn ways of creating an image of wellness and reducing the harmful effects of stress by "self-soothing." Pain has a strong psychological element and so you can practice ways of reducing pain and discomfort. You can also foster positive expectations about medical treatment and your body's ability to heal.

Sleep is often disturbed by stress and we develop unhelpful patterns of behavior which can make it difficult to get deep rest at night. This chapter also includes tips on sleep hygiene and ways of changing thoughts and feelings around sleep. Finally, you can learn how to use the natural dream state to get off to a good night's sleep.

Chapter 6: Setting Goals and Boosting Motivation

How often have you felt the frustration of promising yourself that you <u>will</u> make a change, whether starting a new routine or achieving something important to you, only to find yourself a few months down the line having not achieved those things, *again*? Our basic human needs to feel in control of our lives, to learn and feel challenged, and have a sense of achievement are all assaulted by this sense of failure. If it is continually repeated, life can start to feel "stuck," empty or even meaningless. It is for this important reason that we have devoted this chapter to achieving goals. In this section, you will find an opportunity to stand back and refocus on what is important in your life. You can then learn how to set realistic and achievable goals, and most importantly, how to motivate yourself to achieve them. Rather than floating aimlessly through life, you will have gained some practical skills to begin moving in just the right direction for you.

Chapter 7: Enhancing Assertiveness, Self-esteem, and Confidence

There is a wealth of self-help material available for people who feel they are lacking in self-esteem and confidence, which is perhaps an indication of what a common complaint this is. Trying to feel better about ourselves can prompt us to go down all sorts of unhelpful avenues and sometimes this can lead to unhealthy or destructive habits, which we address in Chapter 8. This chapter will help you take effective steps to becoming a more confident person, starting by cultivating a sense of achievement, which meets an important emotional need in all of us. It goes on to distil some of the best, evidence-based techniques and tools around, providing a practical guide to feeling better about yourself and behaving more assertively. Acting confidently, setting boundaries and saying what you mean may feel unfamiliar and challenging. Don't worry, there are tips along the way that will help you take easy steps so that you can start becoming a more confident person.

Chapter 8: Changing Unhelpful Habits and Patterns

When we are depleted, through excessive stress, traumatic events, loneliness, or boredom, we all have the potential to reach out for destructive "quick fixes." The common ground with any habits is that they give an initial rush of chemical-induced pleasure within the brain. However, these positive feelings are shortly followed by feelings of regret, self-loathing, and a dramatic drop in mood. We are all drawn to different habits; some us will be drawn to an instant chemical hit from alcohol, caffeine, drugs, or food; some of us will use the comfort or even the pain of repetitive nail-biting or skin-picking/cutting to induce the soothing hit of natural endorphins; some of us may behave in ways that temporarily get our emotional need for attention or love met, like shopping beyond our means or sex with strangers. This section is focused on helping you "take the high road" away from behaviors that you know are not working for you, however alluring they seem at the time. It introduces a cycle of change which helps you to understand how to change and how to avoid the danger of self-sabotage. You will be able to identify your "point of no return" in habitual behaviors and then move away from it. Finally, you can learn how to develop a more compassionate approach to your habit, which avoids the emotions of shame, blame, and self-criticism, which in themselves can be overwhelming. These models and techniques will help you to finally leave old habits behind and develop healthy and productive ways of coping with whatever life throws your way.

Chapter 9: Toward Contentment

This final section helps you to put the icing onto the cake of well-being. Having explored how to use the mind to recover and improve well-being in a number of key ways, you can turn your attention to what you want and how you wish to feel as you move forward in your life. Much of this chapter is based on positive emotions as the key to building resilience and a lifetime of well-being. This includes how to develop positive emotions about the future, through cultivating optimism, positive emotions about the past, through gratitude and forgiveness, and positive emotions about the present, through using your signature strengths and enjoying the benefits of getting into **flow**. Finally, we all have the opportunity of connecting our "inner spirit" with our outer world, in terms of discovering a meaning and purpose in life. Paying attention to this need for connection can enhance our mental and physical health and completes the "circle" of well-being. It enables us to give out and connect with others, appreciate the beauty in the world and continue to be curious about our well-being and our very existence.

We hope you enjoy the journey.

Starting out

While you can start looking through the questions, answers and activities in this book in any order, we would encourage you to begin with some fundamentals which we have organized into Chapter 1. These are designed to calm, relax, and focus you. Many of the techniques introduced in this book work most effectively when you are in a relaxed state because your mind is then best able to problem solve, see things in perspective, and access a whole host of unconscious resources which you may not even know are there! You may want to begin by discovering what it is like to be deeply relaxed on a regular basis, and how this can help you to tackle issues which you might want to address. If a particular activity or technique requires that you begin by relaxing, you will be pointed to one of these preliminary exercises first. You can also practice deep relaxation techniques by accessing the recordings on the accompanying CD-ROM.

A note of warning

This guide is not intended to replace seeking medical or professional help for significant physical, emotional, or mental problems. We would suggest that this is essential if you are experiencing any of the following:

- Undiagnosed pain, physical symptoms, or sleep problems
- Symptoms of depression, such as loss of motivation, loss of appetite, changes in sleeping habits, persistent negative thinking
- High levels of anxiety, anger, and recurring panic attacks
- Substance misuse or self-harming behaviors
- Social isolation due to severe lack of confidence or self-esteem

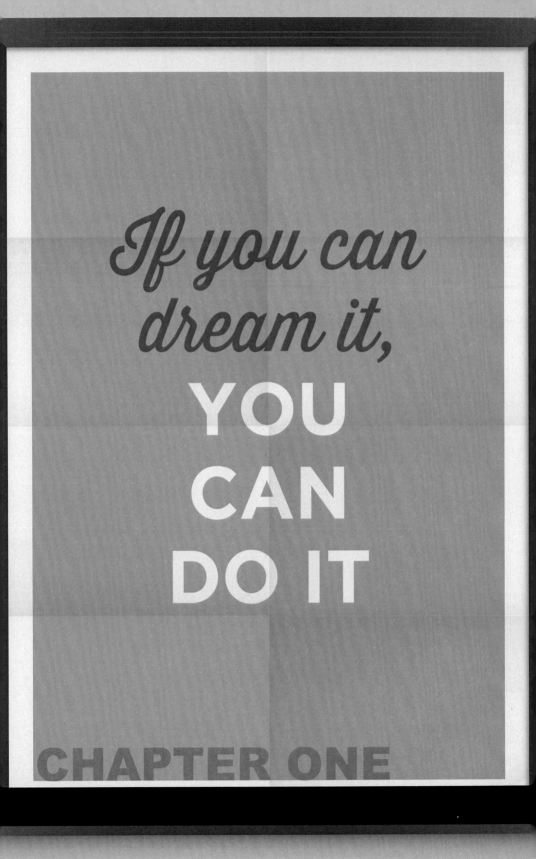

Laying the Foundations of Emotional Health and Well-Being

1. What is the key to emotional health and well-being?

Over the past sixty years the field of psychology has grown into a respected science and we have seen innumerable, different theories about how we think, feel and act, all of which suggest that they have the answers to our mental health. It's no wonder that many of us make confused and unsuccessful attempts at finding happiness and don't know where to turn for effective help. Two UK-based research psychologists and psychotherapists, Joe Griffin and Ivan Tyrrell, founders of the **Human Givens** approach, were indeed puzzled by the plethora of psychological theories, particularly when compared with, for instance, biological theory, where there is one accepted model of how the human body works. With this confusion in mind, Griffin, Tyrrell, and colleagues set about a research project spanning many years, which put under the microscope all available psychological theory and techniques relating to mental well-being. Their aim was to draw together an evidence-based list from these many sources, one which could inform us as humans, what it is we need in our lives to be emotionally well. The resulting list of emotional needs[1] are:

- Security
- The giving and receiving of attention
- Control
- Being part of a wider community
- Privacy
- Intimacy
- Emotional connection with others
- Status

- Achievement
- Meaning and purpose in life

This can provide a definitive checklist that you can refer to, noting where your scores are low and making adjustments in your life accordingly. It can be particularly useful in times of change (e.g., when you have moved house, changed job, or a relationship has ended). This is when we are particularly vulnerable, as our usual ways of getting our needs met may be compromised and we need to be creative about how to get them met in new ways.

Exercise 1. Rate how well your own needs are currently met

2. What is the fight-or-flight response?

Learning to control one of the most basic and vital, underlying factors in our physical and mental health is essential to long-term well-being, and many of the sections in this book are designed to help you prevent or counter what is commonly known as the **"fight-or-flight" response** or stress response.

The human brain is hard-wired for survival. The **amygdala** is part of the limbic system (the "emotional brain") and is involved in many of our emotions and motivations, particularly those that are related to survival. Picture this as a burglar alarm in your house. While you are sleeping soundly, it constantly scans your environment for signs of danger, based on the sensory memories of your past experiences. If it recognizes a threatening *sound*—a loud crash, *sight*—a looming shadow, *sensation*—crawling on the skin, or other sign of danger, it will activate. This will occur before you have had time to investigate whether a burglar has broken in or an overnight guest has decided to go downstairs for a drink of water!

When the alarm is activated, powerful hormones, including **adrenaline**, are released throughout the body, prompting a whole host of physiological changes to enable you to either fight or flee the danger. At this point, you may notice your heart palpitating, your body shaking and sweating and your breath coming in gasps, because your whole body has been mobilized for action. The survival mechanism is firmly based on "live first and ask questions later!"

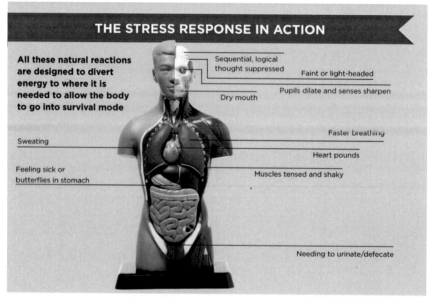

THE STRESS RESPONSE IN ACTION

All these natural reactions are designed to divert energy to where it is needed to allow the body to go into survival mode

Sequential, logical thought suppressed

Faint or light-headed

Dry mouth

Pupils dilate and senses sharpen

Faster breathing

Sweating

Heart pounds

Feeling sick or butterflies in stomach

Muscles tensed and shaky

Needing to urinate/defecate

▲ FIGURE 1.1 The fight-or-flight (stress) response in action

3. How does the fight-or-flight response affect emotional health and well-being?

Unfortunately, the **fight-or-flight response** can "kick off" in a whole range of situations which we associate with fear but which are not, in themselves, life-threatening, for example, being faced with unreasonable work demands, giving a public performance, going into a hospital, or even when we just *imagine* ourselves in uncomfortable situations. The effects may impair our ability to control our body, for example, when we find ourselves shaking and sweating as we walk onto a stage to speak publicly.

Feeling stressed also means that we are more prey to our emotions which operate from a "threat or no-threat," "good or bad" perspective. As the temperature rises, the emotional brain hijacks the higher neocortex (the "thinking brain") which normally provides a more intelligent analysis of what is happening, following the initial danger trigger. Consequently, we find ourselves unable to think clearly, keep things in perspective and make good judgments. For example, we may feel threatened in a meeting, and as our level of upset or anger increases, we are unable to make the fine distinctions we need to analyze and calmly influence opinions in the room.

When we are highly stressed, our anxiety may "spill over" into a full-blown panic attack and we then experience more extreme physiological and mental effects (Q.11).

If we do not allow our bodies to recover and rebalance, long term stress hormones like cortisol are released. In time, these can negatively affect our health, impairing our immune system, digestion, sleep and sex drive, or paving the way into depression, generalized anxiety, or other mental difficulties.

We all need an optimum level of stress to be able to perform effectively when we need to, and sometimes we need the extra emotional arousal to give a big performance. However, being able to "switch off" the fight-or-flight response and "switch on" the body's relaxation response (see Q.5) avoids a build-up of stress hormones and is essential to our well-being—physically, mentally, and emotionally. Stress and relaxation are two sides of the same coin, linked as they are to the two different branches of the central nervous system. We can't experience feelings of relaxation and tension at the same time.

If you feel your stress levels rising, focus the mind on a repetitive task for a minute or two, like counting backward from 300 in threes. This distracts away from thoughts which may be fueling anxiety. Alternatively, take some vigorous exercise which uses the bodily changes which occur with the fight-or-flight response for the purpose they were intended!

4. How can I "switch off" the fight-or-flight response?

When we get stressed, we begin to breathe in short gasps. If we don't take any physical action, for example, running away or fighting for "survival," then we take in more oxygen than we can use. As it is breathed out again, it takes carbon dioxide, essential to the absorption of oxygen by the body, with it. If too much carbon dioxide is lost from the body, we begin to experience the terrifying feeling of suffocating or choking, even though we are still breathing.

One of the quickest ways to stop the **fight-or-flight response** from escalating is to focus on a rhythm of breathing called "7/11 breathing." This stimulates the parasympathetic nervous system which is the part of the central nervous system which enables us to calm down and relax.

Breathe in (preferably through the nose) for a count of seven. Then breathe out more slowly to a count of eleven. The longer exhale stimulates the body's natural relaxation response and quickly stops any panicky feelings. If you can't extend the exhale for eleven, try breathing in to a count of three, and out, more slowly, to a count of five. Alternatively, just hold your breath while you continue counting and then take the next inhalation.

Do this about ten to twenty times, telling yourself that you are relaxing more with each breath.

Concentrate on the counting and notice how much less tense you feel in your body and mind.

In a small number of cases, anxiety symptoms can be triggered by a physical condition, such as thyroid disorder or heart irregularity, or by a sudden change in consumption of caffeine, alcohol, or tranquilizers.

Track 1. "7/11 breathing and body scan"

The **relaxation response** is the "opposite" of the **fight-or-flight response** described in Q.2 and can be prompted by deep relaxation. There are untold benefits to practicing relaxation on a regular basis. Not only does relaxation allow the body a chance to recharge and repair, but it calms the mind so that we are more resourceful in how we handle situations, relate to others, and make decisions. It is a foundation stone for well-being on all levels.

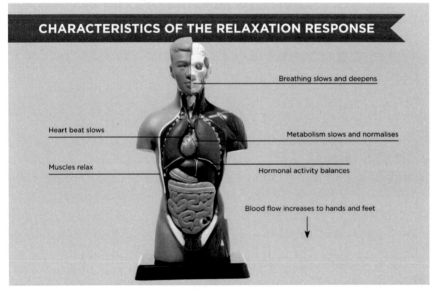

CHARACTERISTICS OF THE RELAXATION RESPONSE

Breathing slows and deepens

Heart beat slows

Metabolism slows and normalises

Muscles relax

Hormonal activity balances

Blood flow increases to hands and feet

▲ FIGURE 1.2 Characteristics of the relaxation response

If you can create one part of this relaxation response, for example, slowing and deepening your breathing, then the chain of other responses will follow.

6. How can I learn to relax?

There are many techniques for prompting the relaxation response, and these are just some of the main ones. It is a good idea to build relaxation into your daily schedule by taking a fifteen to twenty minute break at a regular time of the day which fits in with your routine. This gives the mind and body a chance to recuperate and boosts energy for the rest of the day.

1) Breathing and body scan

Slowing down your breathing, particularly in the 7/11 ratio explained in Q.4, can be helpful as the first step toward relaxation. Following this, you can do a "body scan," bringing your focus to each part of your body in turn (starting with the face and head, and working down to the feet), noticing any tension and then mentally inviting it to release.

Track 1. "7/11 breathing and body scan"

ON THE CD

2) Mindfulness meditation

We can harness the mind to lead the body into deep relaxation, and many activities in this book are designed to help you to do this. **Mindfulness** meditation is a relaxation approach which gently focuses the mind on moment-by-moment experience, for example, on the *breath* entering and leaving the nostrils, or on each *part of the body* in turn, or on *sounds* as they occur in our surroundings. Training our attention to focus in this way, without trying to change anything, brings us fully into the present, away from worries about the past or unhelpful imaginings about the future. **Mindfulness-based stress reduction (MBSR)**—an internationally accepted therapeutic approach developed by Jon Kabat-Zinn[2] at the University of Massachusetts Medical Center in the US—has clinically proven benefits for people with depression, anxiety disorders, and chronic pain.[3]

One way of cultivating mindfulness is to choose a routine activity you do every day, like brushing your teeth, taking a shower, leaving or entering the house, or eating a meal. Each time you do it, bring your full awareness to the activity, moment by moment as best you can. For example, when you wash the dishes, notice every movement your hands and arms make as they scrub and wipe, the shine on the plate, the sound of water sloshing in the bowl, and without judgement, dwell in the mode of being.

PRACTICAL TIP

The CD contains several different mindfulness meditations and an audio recorded track for mindful breathing.

Exercise 2. Mindfulness meditations and Track 2. "Mindful breathing."

3) Visualization

Throughout this book, you will find ideas and suggestions based on the practice of visualization. One of our most powerful mental resources we have as humans is imagination. We can use it to good effect, as when we imagine positive, fulfilling outcomes, or to bad effect, for example, when we imagine all kinds of future catastrophes and fuel our anxiety.

Positive visualization is a wonderful tool which utilizes our imaginations to effect all kinds of changes in how we feel. We can use it to work toward a goal by visualizing the process for achieving success, for example, imagining going to the gym and exercising to get fit, or imagining the immune system seeking and destroying cancer cells. We can also use it to create mental pictures of the goal or result as if it had already occurred, for example, imagining what it is like to be that new, strong, healthy person full of energy and stamina.

The art of visualization is to use all your senses, not just "seeing," but hearing, smelling, and tasting, and feeling textures, movement, and sensations. We all have a dominant sense, but it is helpful to practice using others until your visualization becomes a richer and richer experience.

Visualization focuses the attention inward, creating a deeply relaxing, *trance* state. Trance is a natural state which we all dip into when we daydream, meditate, jog, or otherwise become absorbed in our inner thoughts and experiences. It is sometimes called the **REM** (rapid eye movement) or *programing state* (which also occurs when we dream at night). When we access REM, we create powerful images and we are open to new learning. Using this language of the unconscious mind to make requests for change and to rehearse those changes through guided imagery (visualization), is a foundation of **hypnotherapy**.

As a first step, we can use visualization to create a healthy state of deep relaxation:

Exercise 3. A staircase to relaxation and Track 3. "Step down."

ON THE CD

The CD-ROM contains a script for relaxation visualization and also an audio recorded track for "stepping down" into relaxation.

7. How can I start improving my health and well-being?

Meeting your emotional needs and learning how to relax—both of which we have covered above and will return to throughout the book—are the starting points to making improvements in your health and well-being. While the remainder of the book will help you to tackle different aspects of your overall well-being, learning how to focus on what you <u>do</u> want, tap into your internal resources and utilize what is around you, are other important keys to making improvements across the board.

1) Focusing on what you <u>do</u> want

"The Law of Attraction" was first described by <u>William Walker Atkinson</u>, a very influential figure in the early days of the New Thought Movement, in 1906.[4] Scientists and psychologists who are interested in why certain people succeed in life while others do not, have written prolifically about this psychological phenomenon.

It certainly seems that people who are generally successful in life (that is, they achieve what they set out to achieve) often spend time and energy really focusing on what it is they want. They have a clear vision of how they would like things to be, and once the outcome is achieved, what that will look like, including the ways in which it will differ from the present. This means they know when they have done what they have set out to do, and when it is time to move onto the next step.

The reason business coaches often advise owners of fledgling business to write a business plan, is underpinned by the law of attraction. Once a budding entrepreneur has developed a clear vision of how they want their business to grow and develop, they have attuned their consciousness to noticing opportunities, products, people, and other resources that will support that vision. It is the same process as when you are weighing up whether to buy a new red hatchback, and suddenly notice red hatchbacks everywhere on the road. They were always there, of course, but now you have "tuned in" your consciousness to notice them. This can also be explained by understanding how the brain works in terms of noticing or not noticing. The structure of the brain which is the gatekeeper to awareness is the **reticular formation**. It scans input from the environment, looking out for what is important for survival or relevant to us. Being clear about our vision and goals harnesses and guides the reticular activation process, just as the Law of Attraction suggests.

PRACTICAL TIP

Your imagination is your "reality generator," so learn to use it wisely! Make sure your attention is focused on what you want more of in your life. There are plenty of exercises throughout this book which show you how to harness the power of your imagination in order to achieve changes. When you decide to make a change in your life, however big or small, a key rule is to make sure you spend some time really visualizing what that will be like (follow the guidelines in Exercise 3 on the CD-ROM). For instance, if you want to give up smoking, visualize yourself glowing with health, smelling fresh and clean, and wearing beautiful clothes that you could purchase with all the money you will have saved. Then any time you are tempted to fall back into a habit, you can bring this image to mind and ideally accompany it with a statement to yourself which further embeds the change you are making like, "I am saying no to cigarettes because my health and happiness are now my focus."

The Law of Attraction can, of course, be used to our great detriment if we focus our attention on things we **do not want**. If we are feeling overwhelmed and sad, we can allow our emotional brain to take over and start imagining everything going wrong. For instance, when a long term relationship breaks up and we are feeling bereft, we might think, "I will never meet anyone new, I am so boring and unattractive . . ." If we continue to focus on those feelings, we do become boring by going on about everything that's wrong and that in itself is pretty unattractive! It's no wonder that people will start avoiding us.

Exercise 4. Reality generator

ON THE CD

2) Identifying your resources

Whenever we feel overwhelmed with emotion, we can lose sight of all the good things in our lives, including the strengths and resources we have at our disposal to make positive changes. These include the strengths within us (our qualities, skills, talents, experiences, etc.) and also around us (our friends, family, community, and other support systems which help us access what we need). Psychologists often refer to these as "internal" and "external" resources.

It often seems that at the very time we most need these resources, we are most likely to forget about them. This is because when we feel stressed or overwhelmed our "thinking" brain shuts down (Q.3) and then we can easily feel "all at sea" without a crew or oars! Given the way our brains function, it can be much more helpful to tune into our resources when we feel relatively relaxed and able to recognize them. If we leave it until we slip into the grip of negative thinking and emotions, we may end up believing thoughts such as, "I have no real friends," or "Nothing I have ever done has been successful." Then we <u>really</u> feel un-resourced and this can fuel the negative cycle of depressive thinking which we cover in detail in Chapter 3.

It is a helpful practice to write down our internal and external resources, so that we can refer to them when we are feeling stressed, emotional, or in need Exercise 5. Recognize and use what is good

of support. You can find an exercise for doing this on the accompanying CD-ROM.

CASE STUDY

Kimberley was a fifty-six year old woman who had lost her husband to a heart attack a year earlier. She felt alone and couldn't seem to summon up the energy or motivation to do anything enjoyable. She felt generally anxious about her health and what would happen to her as she grew older and was unable to cope.

Working through the list of emotional needs (Q.1, Exercise 1), Kimberley scored very low on "giving attention" and on "having a meaning and purpose in life."

Next, looking at her resources (Q.7, Exercise 5), Kimberley identified that she had some important external resources available to her—her family—and time to do things. She also pinpointed some of her internal strengths, including liking to help people in practical ways and her playfulness.

She realized that she had neglected to keep in contact with her adult children and that she could give them some attention, by way of offering to look after her two grandchildren on a regular basis. She enjoyed seeing her grandchildren, as she loved to play with them and think up creative ways of keeping them amused. Offering to spend more time with them might fulfill her need to "give attention," as well as "having a meaning and purpose in life." Before her husband died, she had been actively involved in a woodland project to maintain a beautiful piece of woodland near her home. This had given her a sense of belonging and meaning. She felt she might be ready to return to the project.

Kimberley set aside some time for learning to relax and began to build in a ten minute mindful breathing practice each day (Q.6, Exercise 2). She found that it calmed her mind and she was able to see her life as having more possibilities. Going back to the woodland project and spending some time with her grandchildren quickly led to making some new contacts and taking up further interests. She no longer felt a victim of circumstance, but able to enjoy her life, without worrying about the future.

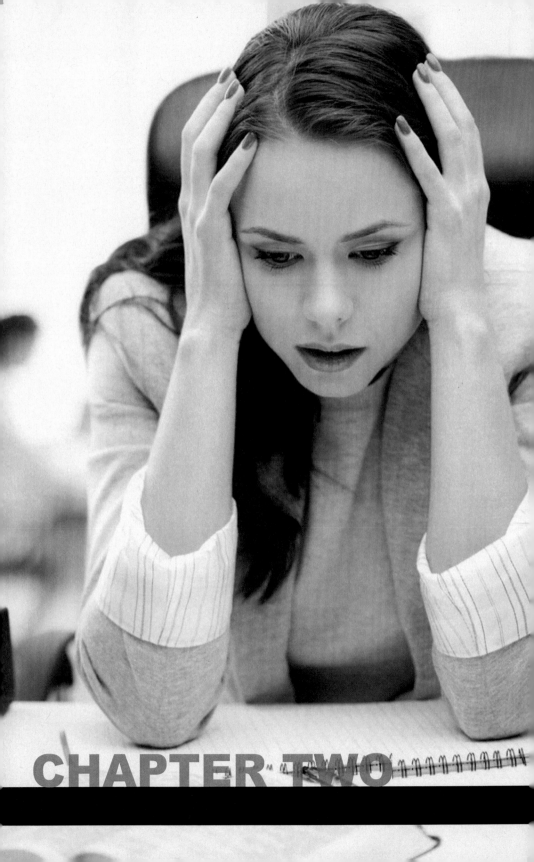

CHAPTER TWO

Dealing with Stress, Anxiety, Panic, and Worry

8. How can I reduce the stress in my life?

How often do you catch yourself saying things like:

> "If only Dad would be kinder/listen to me/have more time for the kids!'
>
> "Why does she behave like that? It's wrong, why doesn't she realize it?'
>
> "People are so racist; they have to realize that they are hurting people. It's terrible!'
>
> "The government doesn't care about the little people, we can't change anything!"
>
> "My boss never listens to me, there's no point in even trying to talk to him!"

And, how does it make you feel when you say something like this, either to yourself or others? Angry? Frustrated? Powerless?

Allowing yourself to focus on what other people are doing wrong and how it should be different is a dead-end path that only leads to misery—*for you*. The culprits of the behavior that you don't like will remain completely unaffected by your thoughts, while your stress levels go up and up!

Exercise 6. Direct your energy to where it can be transformational

ON THE CD

The key to reducing stress is to focus on the things you can do something about, and then to learn ways to calm down in the face of the things you can't.

Interestingly, one of the most effective ways of helping others to change is to change the way <u>you</u> behave. If you let go of trying to change someone else, they will pick up on that shift. They may notice that you no longer make negative comments, or even that you have stopped unconsciously sighing when they do something you don't like. However, remember that it is still possible this won't shift their behavior if they are not ready to change (see "Cycle of change" in Q.45 for more information). Either way, giving another person time and non-judgmental space to change is far more effective than nagging, which can have the opposite effect. Of course you also have the power to remove yourself from people behaving in ways you don't like or to limit contact with people who are making you unhappy. You could consider using these strategies to address items on your list referring to other people.

 You might like to focus on different areas of your life (e.g., relationships, work, leisure, domestic matters). Work out what stresses you in each area, then hone in on what you can actually change and what you have to accept or let go of.

9. How can I calm down in stressful situations?

Anxiety is made up of physical sensations, emotions and thoughts, all of which we can learn to master and calm. Cultivating a sense of calm means that we are functioning in an optimal way. We are physically relaxed, able to step back from our own and others' emotions and can make the best decisions about how we want to respond.

 Think of a calm person you know. What is it about them that exudes a sense of calm? How do they look, how do they move, what do they say, what is their tone of voice, etc.?

We have already described some ways of learning to relax in Chapter 1, including a method of "emergency breathing" which will help you to quickly calm down in difficult situations, and some methods of relaxation which will bring your stress levels down in the longer term.

Resource anchoring is an additional, powerful technique for calming down from the world of **Neuro-linguistic**

programing or NLP. We can learn to set up an "anchor" which triggers a state of calm. An anchor is a sensory trigger which becomes associated with a particular response or state. On a simple level, the sight of a red traffic light prompts us to stop. However, we respond unconsciously to anchors all the time, to both good and bad effect, for example, when the warmth of a sunny morning prompts us to feel good, or the smell of a hospital makes us feel nervous or even sick. The association is strengthened by repetition and by the level of emotion that accompanies it. We can learn how to create our own anchor to elicit the desired state of calm in difficult situations, using the guidelines in Exercise 7.

Exercise 7. Get anchored and Track 4. "An anchor for calm"

ON THE CD

10. How can I control constant worrying?

Reducing the time spent worrying can lower your stress levels and improve your health. Worrying involves a constant repetition of thoughts which lead nowhere. Whereas thinking leads to action and hopefully, relief, worrying about real or imaginary problems triggers the **fight-or-flight response** and raises the levels of stress hormones in our bodies (see Q.1). Continual worrying about something which cannot be resolved can lead to **rumination** which is a major feature of depression (Q.21).

Worrying can take two forms: "real worries" based on real-life situations, and unfounded worries based on the imagination. Each can be dealt with in slightly different ways.

Worrying about real-life issues needs to be kept in its place as a first step to tackling any problems in a resourceful way. A cognitive behavioral therapy (**CBT**) approach is to allocate "worry time" which is clearly ring-fenced, for example, twenty minutes at a particular time of day.[5] Having a set place to worry or even a "worry chair" can help to delineate this time even more. For the rest of the day, we can try to detract away from the first signs of worrying, knowing that our worry time will come! During worry time, we should do nothing except worry. In practice, although this can be quite challenging, it can sometimes help to put worry into perspective.

Unfounded worries can be based on anxiety-fuelling beliefs, for example, imagined illnesses, or superstition. Our powerful imaginations can take us into all kinds of future disasters. Through deep relaxation, we can learn to think about the worry while feeling relaxed and without emotion.

 PRACTICAL TIP Learn to realistically evaluate future "threats." Rate from one to ten how likely it is to happen. What is the very worst that could happen? What is the best that could happen? The likelihood is that the reality will fall somewhere in between.

Dealing with unfounded worries might require specialist help, for example, from a CBT therapist or hypnotherapist.

Here are a few further tips about managing worrying:

- Understand your worry patterns. How do they start, what comes next, how do they end? Recognizing the pattern gives you an opportunity to regain control and change it.

- Check whether you are meeting your basic emotional needs (see Q.1), and are getting enough sleep (see Q.33).

- Laughter is a natural medicine for dissolving worry and anxiety, without side effects! Watch funny films, ask friends to e-mail good jokes or funny stories, and spend time with people who like to laugh.

- Learn to relax deeply, which helps you to take a step back from worries, come up with solutions and see the bigger picture (see Q.6).

- Use **mindfulness** practice to turn off busy and worrisome thoughts (see Q.6, Exercise 2).

Exercise 8. Worry time

ON THE DVD

Approaches which combat negative thinking will also help to reduce worrying (see Chapter 3.)

11. What causes panic attacks?

A panic attack is the same as the body's normal fear reaction, but it is happening inappropriately, that is, in an ordinary situation. As we saw in Q.2, our essential survival mechanism, the **fight-or-flight response,** can begin to kick off at times when we don't need it to. This stress response can catch us unawares and tip us into an experience of panic.

This can happen for several reasons. The **limbic brain,** which stores sensory memory, may have learned to associate features of our surroundings with danger, because they were present at a time when we experienced a high degree of fear or trauma in the past. These features in themselves might be entirely non-threatening, for example, a harmless spider, a crowded or confined space, or the smell of a hospital ward. However, they have become associated with the feeling of being in danger, and this "pattern matching" is at the heart of both panic attacks and phobias.

Panic attacks can also arise from the misuse of our powerful imaginations. Just imagining all kinds of disaster scenarios, for example, when we misinterpret bodily symptoms and convince ourselves that we have an incurable illness, can escalate our levels of fear until we trigger the fight-or-flight response—even though there is nothing dangerous in the present. Thirdly, our level of stress might be so high that a further challenge pushes our anxiety over the edge—the straw that breaks the camel's back.

Other factors which may prompt a panic attack include:

* toxins or chemicals in our system, for example, caffeine or some drugs
* negative thinking and worrying

- anger, rage, and other intense emotions
- accident and injury
- piling pressure on ourselves (a good example being the "**adrenaline** junkie")

The physical symptoms which mobilize our bodies to get out of danger (see Q.2) can be frightening to experience at times when there is nothing to run away from and no one to fight. Escalating blood pressure, pounding heart, and quick, shallow breathing may be accompanied by shaking in the limbs and tingling or numbness in the arms and hands as blood flow and oxygen go to the big muscles. We may feel sick, experience chest pain, or even feeling we are choking. Panic attacks are often accompanied by extreme thoughts:

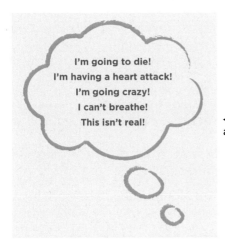

◄ FIGURE 2.1 Thoughts accompanying a panic attack

We can take the power out of these thoughts by countering them with helpful thoughts such as, "I've been in this situation before," "If I breathe slowly, I know it will pass."

Hold your breath for up to fifteen seconds to avoid hyperventilation, before resuming calm, slower breathing or 7/11 breathing (Q.4). Remember that panic attacks cannot harm you and usually last for no longer than ten minutes, even if allowed to follow their normal course. However, it is important to seek professional advice if you are experiencing repeated attacks.

12. How can I learn to overcome rising anxiety, worry, and panic attacks?

Practicing relaxation or 7/11 breathing (see Chapter 1) can help us to notice what we are feeling and thinking and to "stand back" and observe our thoughts and worries. We can then make a judgment about how useful (or not) they are.

Remember this acronym to help distract away from worry and anxiety: S stands for "Stop!" O stands for "Observe" and S for "Steer away."

PRACTICAL TIP

Once we notice that we are engaging in unproductive worrying or imaginings, we can then distract ourselves and break the pattern.

There are several techniques for learning to avoid or overcome rising anxiety and to shorten the cycle of symptoms, should a panic attack occur.

1) Distraction

Many of us who tend to get anxious or worry find it difficult to stop, once our **fight-or-flight response** is activated.

Different distracting activities work better for different people, but these could include:

- Get in touch with other people, for example, by phoning a friend
- Walk briskly around the block or the garden
- Spend a couple of minutes using 7/11 breathing (Q.4)
- Write down the thoughts you're having and test out the evidence for them (Q.20)
- Listen to a relaxation recording
- Do some housework
- Do some vigorous exercise (e.g., star jumps, running up and down stairs)
- Count backward from 300 in threes (this engages the rational, thinking part of the brain)

• Mow the lawn, bake a cake of do something else you can enjoy, and get absorbed in.

Even practicing one of the above for as little as thirty seconds can help to break the chain of thoughts and physiological responses which can spiral into panic or a bout of worrying.

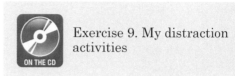

Exercise 9. My distraction activities

2) The AWARE technique

Staying in a difficult situation by using the AWARE technique "tells" the **amygdala** that you are safe and that there is no need to fight or run away. This can give you a vital sense of getting back in control and can weaken unhelpful associations between the situation and the alarm trigger.

Exercise 10. The AWARE technique

3) Grading

This approach can be useful if you are avoiding particular situations which make you anxious, or in tackling phobias (see p. 26). It involves deliberately changing your behavior and going back into difficult situations, in a step-by-step way.

Exercise 11. Anxiety grading

4) Long-term strategies

Panic attacks (and high levels of stress) arise from a spiralling cycle of physical symptoms, thoughts, emotions, and actions. These can be avoided by learning new skills: reducing *physical symptoms* by learning relaxation and controlled breathing (see Chapter 1); reducing *emotional* and *mental symptoms* by tackling worry, negative thinking and anger (see Chapters 3 and 4); and *changing behavior* so that you can act resourcefully in challenging situations.

In order to change behavior, you may want to make changes to your lifestyle, by ensuring that you are meeting your emotional needs (see Q.1), reducing sources of stress (see Q.8), setting goals (see Chapter 6), and breaking unhelpful habits (see Chapter 8).

There are a number of other high anxiety states which are briefly described below, along with psychological treatments which can help.

13. What is a phobia and how can it be treated?

"A phobia may be defined as a marked or persistent fear that is excessive, unreasonable, or out of proportion to the danger that the situation or object presents."[6]

As with panic attacks, phobias involve both psychological and physical symptoms of anxiety, and a strong drive to escape the situation or object. We can develop a phobia for just about anything from specific objects, such as bridges, spiders or buttons, and specific situations, such as flying, heights, or vomiting, to more complex situations like social phobias (a fear of being "exposed" to unfamiliar people in a variety of situations) or agoraphobia (an avoidance of situations and places where there is no obvious means of "escape" and which leads to a general fear of going out). Sometimes phobias develop where the person has experienced a traumatic event and the object or situation which was present at that time becomes associated with the high emotional arousal they experienced. Subsequent exposure to that object or situation (even where it was not the cause of the original trauma) triggers the **fight-or-flight response** leading to a strong feeling that the individual is in danger.

Psychological treatments include:

1) Systematic desensitization

Developed by Dr Joseph Wolpe,[7] this form of behavior therapy is based on findings that many fears can be seen as learned responses. It involves "graded exposure," based on developing a hierarchy of images in relation to the object or situation, with items graded in terms of the level of fear experienced. The individual is then taught a new response which is incompatible with fear (deep relaxation) in relation to each item, beginning with the "easiest" (lowest fear) and working up to the most difficult. Graded exposure is usually conducted first in the imagination and then in real life, working in small increments toward direct contact with the object or being fully in the most feared situation. For example, if a person has a fear of snakes, the therapist might begin by asking the person to imagine graded situations involving snakes, to showing them a small picture of a snake, to bringing them into a place where there is a real snake behind glass, to finally inviting them to handle a live snake.

2) Cognitive Behavioral Therapy (CBT)

CBT therapists have built on this idea of graduated exposure to the source of fear which enables the person to learn that it is safe to remain in a situation or in contact with the feared object. They address an additional need for people to change their thoughts and memories, not just their behavior, in relation to their phobias and anxiety. CBT usually involves:

- Testing thoughts and beliefs around what might happen in a feared situation, for example, a belief that you might collapse when speaking in public. This enables the person to develop more realistic and supportive ways of thinking.
- Graded exposure to the situation. Anxiety reduces as the person remains in the situation, and also

on repeated exposures. The AWARE and Grading techniques (Q.12) are based on this principle.

Regular relaxation practice (see Chapter 1) and long-term strategies as described for panic attacks in Q.12(4) can also help to reduce anxiety around phobias.

3) Visual/kinesthetic dissociation or rewind technique

Visual/kinesthetic dissociation or "rewind," derived from NLP, is used in clinical **hypnotherapy** to treat phobias and post-traumatic stress disorder. Simply described, the technique works by allowing the individual with a phobia, whilst in a safe relaxed state, to reprocess the memories connected with the phobia. Described in more detail in Q.15, the process distances the person from the normal phobic response and enables the sensory memory to be "shifted" in the brain from the **amygdala** to the **neocortex**, where long-term memories are stored. The fear response is then no longer elicited by the object or situation associated with the phobia. This technique has been found to work quickly and effectively with phobia and is sometimes called "the fast phobia cure."[8]

14. What is a generalized anxiety state?

Sometimes a person can experience frequent and high levels of anxiety and worry as a general condition, and this can have a negative impact on their social, family, and work lives. Although there is no immediate threat to their safety, they may worry unduly about all kinds of thing, such as their health, the future, etc. Generalized anxiety is sometimes triggered by stressful events, and often accompanies phobias. The six central symptoms are:[9]

- restlessness
- being easily fatigued
- difficulty in concentrating or the mind going blank
- irritability

- muscle tension
- sleeplessness

There may also be a general sense of underlying foreboding.

Psychological treatments based on **CBT** and deep relaxation will help to reduce anxiety levels and tackle unhelpful thinking patterns associated with this condition. The person may be taught to deal with real worries through problem solving skills, and unfounded worries by thinking about the worry while deeply relaxed and without emotion. Additionally, any trauma will need to be deconditioned (see **Q.15**).

15. What is PTSD and how can it be treated?

Post-traumatic stress disorder or PTSD can occur when a person has experienced an event outside of the normal range of human experience, in which they felt extreme fear, for example, accidents, emotional and sexual abuse, and war trauma. When there is high "emotional arousal" or fear, the **amygdala** triggers the **fight-or-flight response** to prompt the person to escape from danger or fight for their life. If they are unable to escape from the situation or are overwhelmed with emotion, the fight-or-flight response may continue to fire, even when the event has long finished and they are safe again. A person with PTSD may experience nightmares, vivid memories, or "flashbacks," in which they re-experience the fear that they felt at the time, over and over again. They may also feel constantly anxious and depressed, and experience panic attacks or emotional numbness, in which they are out of touch with their feelings.

High levels of stress hormone caused by the trauma inhibit the higher, thinking part of the brain (the **neo-cortex**) and the **hippocampus** which plays a role in recording memories. When an incident is recalled in a state of low arousal—i.e., absence of fear—the hippocampus re-logs the memory as past and no longer threatening.

Helpful psychological treatments include the following:

1. Visual/kinesthetic dissociation or rewind

Visual/kinesthetic dissociation or rewind treatment, derived from **NLP**, helps the person to separate their fearful feelings from the usually vivid and painful images they have of the original event. This process involves the person watching the old memories on an imaginary screen, while relaxing deeply in a place in their minds that they associate with calm and safety. The memories are disrupted by being played at speed backward and forward on the screen. The person may be invited to imagine floating into the screen and rewinding themselves backward through the memory, just as if they are inside an old, out-of-date movie. The process of watching and rewinding through each memory several times, whilst feeling deeply relaxed and dissociated from the high emotions of the original event, disrupts the associations between the emotional memory and the images, helping the **amygdala** (the "alarm system" in the brain) to register that the person is now safe around these memories, and that they can be "processed" as long-term memories in the **neocortex**.

If appropriate, the individual is then helped to imagine future scenarios in which they stay calm and behave in more resourceful ways. Following rewind treatment, the individual often finds it difficult to summon up the memories of the trauma—the past traumatic images seem to be more vague and distant in time, as with most old memories, and no longer provoke a high level of emotion when thought about.

The advantage of this treatment is that there is no painful revisiting of the original event and the client can feel in control of the process. In addition, the therapist need not know any details of what happened at all, since each memory is only briefly acknowledged and labeled by the client, rather than discussed at length.

2. Eye Movement Desensitization and Reprocessing (EMDR)

EMDR, first discovered by Dr Francine Shapiro, a psychologist at the Mental Research Institute in Palo Alto, California, is a therapy in which rapid-eye movements (REM) are induced while the person focuses on a disturbing memory, image, feeling, or physical sensation associated with the original, traumatic event.[10] These eye movements are similar to naturally occurring dream sleep. One of the functions of dreaming is thought to be processing unresolved emotion or "unfinished business" from the day (Q.21). In a similar way, REM induced by EMDR helps the person to access memories and feelings which they may have not been able to recall, and then work through and "reprocess" these. This can involve taking on board more positive beliefs and thoughts about life, in place of the negative beliefs they automatically took on board at the time of the trauma. For example, a person who had been abused as a child might have been unconsciously living with a belief of being unworthy and unsafe in the world. They might now integrate a new belief that they are safe and deserve to find love and fulfillment in their life.

CBT can also help the sufferer to challenge their thinking around past traumatic events, and longer-term strategies include those already discussed in Q.12.

16. What is OCD and how can it be treated?

Obsessive-Compulsive Disorder or OCD is driven by high anxiety and the need for a sense of safety, security, and control. It can include obsessive and seemingly senseless *thoughts*, such as thoughts about contamination, fears of leaving the cooker on or the door unlocked, or harming others, and compulsive *behavior* which is an attempt to assuage the anxiety and bring order to the person's emotional life, for example, constantly checking, washing, or counting. For example, obsessive thoughts around the fear of contamination can lead to avoiding touching doorknobs, surfaces, and other people, and washing hands over and over again, taking up huge amounts of time and energy.

Psychological therapies for OCD include **CBT** to identify the nature of fearful or guilty thoughts and replace them with more helpful alternatives, and rewind (Q.15) to reduce the high emotional arousal associated with certain situations and behaviors, together with teaching relaxation and deep breathing to reduce anxiety symptoms. As with other anxiety disorders, helping the person to meet their basic human needs for security and control (Q.1) in healthy ways is at the heart of long-term recovery.

CASE STUDY

Bob was a forty year old successful sales executive with a new, high pressure job. He was keen to make a good start and was working hard to exceed his monthly sales targets. He had always seen himself as a bit of a "worrier" and soon began to have doubts about his capacity to fulfill his own expectations at work. One of his sons was getting into trouble at school, and he worried about where this would lead. He began to imagine getting fired from work for failing to meet the targets, not being able to make the mortgage payments on the house, and his son getting expelled from school. He stopped sleeping properly at night, and this meant that he felt dull and couldn't think clearly when he was at work. He knew that he needed to be "sharp thinking" to do his job well and so this just added another pressure. One morning, on his way to work, he began to feel fearful and shaky and had to pull off the road. He could feel his heart pounding and thought he was going to have a heart attack. It took quite a while for him to calm down. He couldn't face going into work that day, and took a day off sick, which he had never done before. It was even harder to get up the next day and go in.

Bob decided to share his worries with his good friend, Harvey, who always seemed to be at ease with his life. Harvey encouraged him to look at the things in his life which were causing him stress. It was true that he set himself targets at home, as well as at work, and some of these were adding to his worries. Bob decided to postpone some of his home-related goals (clearing out the garage, repainting the front of the house), and concentrate his energies on meeting, rather than exceeding, his work targets, something he felt instantly more confident about doing. He talked to his wife about going to a relaxation class together, and taking a morning off so that they could visit their son's teacher and talk through how best to tackle his problems.

Bob began to recognize his worry patterns and to distract away from unhelpful thoughts by going for a brisk walk or mowing the lawn. If he found himself worrying a lot, he learned to postpone his worrying to a time later in the day, when he could sit upstairs for a few minutes by himself. By using his new relaxation and deep breathing skills, he could see how many of his worries were unfounded and that it was more helpful to focus on the things he could change.

Bob started to sleep better and his old confidence in his work abilities returned. He found that he was comfortably juggling work and home life, and spending more time with his sons. He even found time to plan a family vacation.

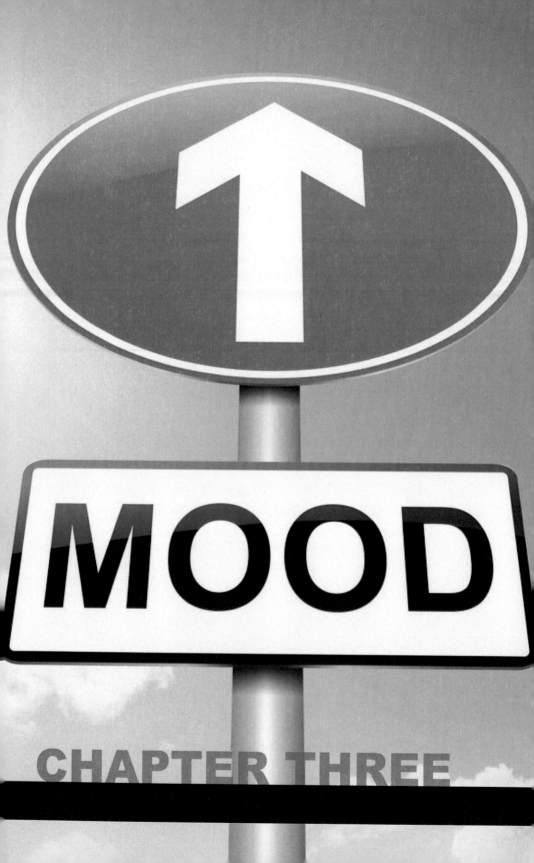

CHAPTER THREE

Controlling Negative Thinking and Avoiding Depression

17. How does negative thinking affect my well-being?

This chapter provides practical steps to taking control of negative thinking—which can be "toxic" to our well-being. This is because negative thoughts can be highly emotionally arousing, triggering the **fight-or-flight response** to perceived danger, or sometimes producing euphoria. Both of these states disable our "thinking brain" and lead us into problematic behavior. Prolonged negative thinking and the resulting triggering of the fight-or-flight response can lead to depression (Q.21) and panic attacks (Q.11) or generalized anxiety (Q.14). It also has a detrimental effect on our physical well-being, making us more prone to illness and disease as it diminishes the effectiveness of the immune system (Q.28 and Q.29).

18. What are the common ways of thinking negatively?

It takes courage to admit to ourselves that we have been slaves to negative thinking, but once we realize that these thoughts are <u>not</u> fact, our lives can turn around. Below is the master list of thinking "errors" that trip us up at times.

As you read through the list, see if you can identify with any of these styles of negative thinking, then <u>be on your guard</u> for when they occur. You might like to name the part of you that can get caught up in these patterns of thinking, so that you can quickly identify when "he" or "she" tries to creep in and ruin your day. For instance, if you are prone to making a mountain out of a mole hill, or "catastrophizing," you might say to yourself, "Uh oh, here comes Catastrophizing Cathy, I had better cross the street away from her so that I can stay in my rational mind!"

Common faulty ways of thinking

Black or white thinking (i.e., it <u>must</u> be one thing or another)

Only seeing a "right" way and a "wrong" way, without allowing any possibilities in between, for example, unless everything is "right," then it's all a total failure (see also Q.22).

Catastrophizing

Jumping to the worst possible conclusion in any given situation, without considering all the other possibilities, for example, you sneeze once and know you are coming down with flu again.

Over-generalizing

Because something has happened once, believing that this will always be the case, for example, you went to a busy restaurant and felt panicky and now you believe that you will always feel this way when you go out to eat.

Focusing on the negative

Ignoring the positives in any situation, for example, feeling devastated and a "failure" that you have lost your job, while ignoring all the ways you have succeeded in life or the resources you still possess, such as having lost jobs before and always having found another (often better) one, having good networks, employable skills, and other areas of your life that are working well.

Jumping to unfounded conclusions

Allowing your imagination to take over and believe the fantasies it comes up with, for example, when a friend makes an off the cuff remark which you take personally and then jump to the conclusion that they no longer like you or want your friendship.

Believing and using controlling statements

Using words like "should," "must," "ought," "never," and "always" mean that we are being controlled by rules that we, or often someone else, have made up for us somewhere along the line. Let these words be warning signs that someone else is doing our thinking for us. They are usually reflections of another person's views that we have unconsciously taken on and that can keep us trapped in fixed and unhelpful ways of living.

19. How can I begin to take control of my negative thinking?

The first and most fundamental skill is to start to become <u>aware</u> of your thoughts. This sounds simple, but we are so conditioned to accept our thoughts as fact, that we often identify with them to the point that we feel we <u>are</u> our thoughts.

By becoming aware of our thoughts, we give ourselves a very powerful tool:

We separate ourselves from our thoughts, so that we can be objective about their accuracy!

This has been called stepping into our **observing self**, a term introduced by psychiatrist Arthur Deikman[11] to explain the part of our mind that "steps back" from the world of thought. It sees what is going on from a more detached perspective, rather than being blindly led by our thoughts as if they were fact.

When you learn to do this and keep doing this, it can be surprisingly liberating. You are no longer a slave to negative thoughts that can depress your mood and stop you moving on in your life. You can realize that thoughts are just thoughts and that you have a <u>choice</u> to not be a slave to negative thoughts (see the "Mindful thoughts" activity in Exercise 2 on the CD-ROM for a way of utilizing the observing self in this way).

20. How can I challenge and reduce negative thinking?

So far, we have emphasized the fact that thoughts are <u>just</u> thoughts, rather than unmovable facts that must be accepted. Thoughts are reflections of your mood, and that mood will affect the perspective you have on what is currently going on in your life and around you.

We all have the power to start noticing our thoughts and consciously change them for the better, so that we have a more balanced and objective perspective. Constructive thoughts are far more helpful to us and will improve our mood. This is not to say that it is easy to change our thoughts; it takes practice and perseverance, but it <u>is</u> possible to harness the power of realistic, helpful thinking, rather than allowing negative thoughts to drag us down and prevent us from achieving our goals. Once you begin to see the results of letting go of negative thinking, you really start to experience how liberating this can be.

Many of the techniques we introduce throughout this book for changing patterns of thinking are based on **cognitive behavioral therapy (CBT)**. Here are two key approaches:

1) Collecting evidence for and against

If you are feeling low or beset with negative thoughts, seeing things more objectively and trying to find evidence against a negative thought can seem difficult. This is because in an emotional state, your brain sometimes discounts the more objective evidence and you can get "locked" into negative thinking. In order to help your brain work more constructively, use 7/11 breathing for a few minutes (Q.4), and then try the activities below.

Imagine that you are advising your best friend (rather than yourself) to look for evidence which supports or counters your thoughts. What would you say to them if they were thinking these thoughts? Looking at your situation from a different viewpoint can help you be more objective and see all the available evidence to counter negative thoughts.

PRACTICAL TIP

Exercise 12. Use basic CBT techniques to take control of your thoughts

ON THE CD

Here is a more detailed activity for challenging negative thinking:

2) Changing controlling "self-talk"

There are certain patterns of thinking that get reflected in what we say to others, and also to ourselves, in the form of controlling "self-talk." Controlling language limits us to "fixed rules" for living, stops us from seeing all the possibilities in life and so prevents us from living optimistically and with joy.

Controlling patterns of thinking and speech nearly always come from our early conditioning, that is, what we were taught as young children about how the world operates, our place within it, and what is "okay" and "not okay." Of course, as children, we accept these assumptions as the absolute truth. However, when we become adults, we may want to start to question some of these assumptions, particularly if they are not helpful to our growth and happiness.

There are three words that many of us use frequently and without question in our day-to-day speech and thoughts, which do not serve us well. These three words tell us that there is only one way to look at life, that things are either right or wrong, and that there are no other possibilities. Of course, there may be rare occasions where that might be true, but generally speaking, it is far more accurate to say that there are many ways of looking at one situation, there are numerous possibilities in life, things are constantly changing, and that it's likely that people will have different opinions.

So, what are these three little "toxic" words? They are:

SHOULD, OUGHT, and MUST!

All three of these words impose fixed rules, they tell us there are no other possibilities, this is how it is and nothing can change. Using them may limit both ourselves and other people we put on the receiving end.

Here are some examples of how they are frequently used:

"I **MUST** always look perfect."
"I **OUGHT** to be better at this."
"I **SHOULD** be 5 pounds lighter."
"I **SHOULD** have passed that test, I am so stupid."
"I still haven't found a loving partner, I **MUST** be unlovable."
"You **OUGHT** to get a more interesting job."

Do you see how by using those words, we close down other perfectly plausible possibilities in any given situation? The person who hasn't found a loving partner, might be looking in the wrong places. <u>Who says</u> you must look perfect all the time? How boring not to just let go sometimes! <u>Who says</u> you must be better at something? You can't be good at everything! So if you want your life to stay stuck, to rob yourself of joy, happiness, and curiosity about life, keep using them!

PRACTICAL TIP

The way out of these fixed rules of language is to <u>question</u> them. Be on guard and every time you hear yourself say one of these words to yourself or others, question it. A really simple and useful way to do this is simply to say, "<u>Who says</u>?" in response to "should," "must," and "ought." They came from somewhere but they just might not be relevant anymore, so maybe it's time to let go of them?

Imagine that there is an "alarm" attached to "should," "must," and "ought." Whenever you catch yourself saying any of those words, picture this alarm ringing loudly in your head, warning you to run a mile from that old conditioning. Give yourself a break and live freely in the here and now.

21. How is negative thinking linked to depression?

The American psychologist, Martin Seligman and colleagues, developed the concept of "learned helplessness" as a way of understanding depression.[12] Arising from observations of animals, they described it as a psychological condition in which a human being or an animal has learned to act or behave helplessly in a particular situation, even when they actually <u>have</u> the power to change an unpleasant or even harmful circumstance.

People who are depressed often feel that they have no control over what happens to them because of the way in which they interpret life's events. Their pessimistic style of thinking means that they tend to see "bad" events as *permanent,* affecting *the whole* of their lives and to do with their own, *personal failings.* On the other hand, "good" events are seen as *temporary*, specific to one part of their lives and to do with *external* circumstances, for example, a "lucky" break. One way out of these patterns of thinking is to use the techniques described in Q.20 and to start looking for small things which you *can* control.

Depression is often characterized by a loss of energy, motivation, and pleasure in day-to-day life and activities. An important factor behind these symptoms is too much negative **rumination**. This happens when we churn around the same hopeless thoughts and are unable to resolve their content through any action. The result is over-arousal of the emotional centers in the **limbic system**, which triggers the **fight-or-flight response** (Q.2) and reduces levels of **serotonin** (the "feel-good" chemical) in the brain.

Research psychologist, Joe Griffin's work at the Human Givens Institute in the UK[13] suggests that when people ruminate in a negative way, they tend to over-dream at night, since a function of REM sleep could be to discharge arousal "left over" from the day, so that the higher **neocortex** can deal with the emotionally arousing situations of the next day. Over-dreaming deprives the sleeper from restful, recuperative deep sleep and this in turn, leads to exhaustion the next morning. No wonder that we feel less inclined to do the things which give us pleasure. We then feel down, ruminate more, dream more, and find ourselves feeling even lower, and so the cycle continues.

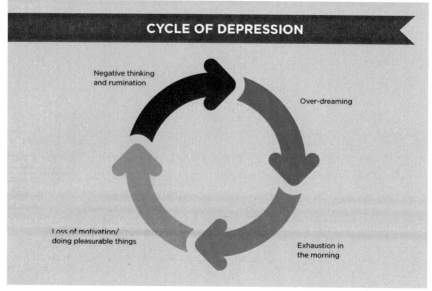

CYCLE OF DEPRESSION

Negative thinking and rumination

Over-dreaming

Exhaustion in the morning

Loss of motivation/ doing pleasurable things

▲ FIGURE 3.1 Cycle of depression

22. How can I avoid the depression cycle?

So how can we avoid getting into this downward cycle of depression? Examining the nature of our rumination can be a starting point.

• Negative thinking

As we saw in Q.21, depression is characterized by a certain style of negative thinking. Use the ideas in this chapter of the book to challenge those thoughts and start creating more hopeful thoughts. Learning to say "Stop!" when you notice a negative thought, and practicing the art of positive thinking is like creating a new, clear pathway in the mind, while allowing the old one to become overgrown and impenetrable.

• Past focus

If rumination is focused on the past and what has gone wrong, it doesn't have to mean that tomorrow will be the same. Changing what you do now will change your future, whereas doing what you always did will mean that you continue to get what you always got. Sometimes we can learn from looking at what we did in the past that worked well for us.

• Guilt

Sometimes there's a guilt factor present, for example, feeling that we are 100 percent to blame for how bad things are, or that we are bad or faulty in some way. If so, we can challenge these thoughts, for example, by asking ourselves what would our partner or best friend say if they heard us making these kinds of statements. How else could we respond in a situation, other than feeling guilty?

• Perfectionism

If perfectionism is a problem, we can ask ourselves whether we are trying to please someone else and give ourselves permission to do things in a less than perfect way.

 PRACTICAL TIP When relaxed, ask yourself how would it be if you were to wake up tomorrow feeling a bit better? What might you be able to do? See yourself in this new scene, looking brighter, and being more active. Float into that new you. How does it feel?

At the same time as exploring our rumination patterns, we can use another technique for breaking down a certain way of thinking which often characterizes depression. People with depression see the world in black and white terms. They use words like "always" or "never," "all" or "nothing," finding it difficult to see the shades of grey between the two extremes. For example, rather than noticing that they feel "a little bit better" today, they may continue to say that they "feel awful" and that "everything is terrible." Increasing our flexibility of thinking gives us back a sense of control and the ability to cope with the ever-present change and uncertainties of life.

Scaling is a simple method of breaking down "all or nothing" thinking that holds problems in place. It engages two powerful aspects of our minds—the thinking brain and

If you tend to make global statements about how you feel, try this practice. Rate how "down" or "low" you feel from zero—as "low" as you could possibly feel, to ten—as good as you could possibly imagine feeling. You could rate at key points in the day, for example, first thing, going to work, before going to bed. As the days go by, notice times when your rating is slightly higher. What are you thinking or doing which is making the difference? Then, do more of these things.

Exercise 13. Use "scaling" to get back in the driver's seat

the ability we have to observe ourselves—to rate different aspects of how we are feeling. We can rate with numbers, shades of a color, a musical scale, weather conditions, or any other system which fills in the two extremes with a gentler continuum of options. This moves us out of anxiety or emotion and into making finer distinctions about our feelings and our progress toward improved well-being.

Finally, in order to look more objectively at our patterns of depressive thinking, we need to take regular, deep relaxation to calm our minds, and put things back in perspective.

23. How do I know whether I'm depressed?

The symptoms of depression can be complex and vary widely among individuals. As we have already seen, depression may be characterized by psychological symptoms such as negative thinking, loss of motivation and pleasure, and feelings of helplessness, sadness, or guilt (Q.21). These psychological symptoms can be severe and include high anxiety, suicidal thoughts, and thoughts of self-harming. Depression may also have physical symptoms like sleep disturbance, loss of energy, and changes in weight or appetite. Social symptoms can include avoiding contact with friends, not going out, neglecting hobbies and interests, and relationship difficulties. While mild depression may have some impact on daily life, moderate or severe depression can have a major impact and be extremely debilitating.

If you experience symptoms of depression for most of the day, every day, for more than two weeks, you should seek help from your physician.

24. How can depression be treated?

The effectiveness of certain forms of psychological therapies has been increasingly recognized in the treatment of depression, and in more severe cases of depression, these are often combined with antidepressant medication, rather than relying on medication alone.

Cognitive behavioral therapy has become a standard treatment for depression in the United Kingdom and elsewhere. Studies have shown that cognitive therapy is as efficacious as antidepressant medication at treating depression, and it seems to reduce the risk of relapse even after its discontinuation.[14] We have already seen how negative thinking patterns are central to depression, and how a cognitive behavioral approach can help the sufferer to challenge hopeless styles of thinking. When this is combined with reducing anxiety and stress through

 Use any of the relaxation practices in Chapter 1. Then, when you are ready, bring your awareness to your thoughts. Notice thoughts as they arise, as they linger in the mind, and as they eventually dissolve and disappear. There is no need to try to control these thoughts in any way. It is as if they are projected onto a film screen and you can just sit, watching the screen, waiting for a thought or image to arise. When it does, attend to it as long as it is there, then let it go as it passes away. If any thoughts bring feelings or emotions, pleasant or unpleasant, just note the strength and nature of these feelings and allow them to be as they are.

If you are repeatedly drawn into the drama of your thinking, bring your focus back to the belly and your breathing, as in Exercise 2 (1) on the CD-ROM. You may then like to try listening to Track 2 "Mindful breathing" on the CD-ROM, or "Mindful thoughts" meditation in Exercise 2.

deep relaxation, the individual can begin to frame their experiences and thoughts in more hopeful ways.

Mindfulness is a powerful practice for both calming the mind and body and for keeping the focus in the present, away from the problems of the past, or the imagined catastrophes of the future (see Q.6). **Mindfulness-based stress reduction (MBSR)** has been shown to help people break out of the downward spiral of mood and prevent the pattern of recurring bouts of depression.[15, 16]

Human Givens therapy

Human Givens therapy integrates behavioral, cognitive, and interpersonal approaches with relaxation and visualization techniques in order to motivate people with depression to widen their life view, raise their self-esteem and solve problems. The Human Givens therapist works alongside patients to address their emotional needs (Q.1) and give practical guidance for breaking problems down into manageable chunks (focusing outward on resolution rather than inward on non-productive worrying). As with CBT, they will use thought and belief challenging to prompt individuals out of their black and white thinking and **reframe** their negative comments in a novel, positive way. They will also set tasks and support the development of new skills to help the individual re-engage with life, for example, through exercising, returning to enjoyable activities, or getting involved in helping others (again, to direct their attention outward).

Above all, the imagination is activated through guided visualization to help individuals vividly see themselves making the changes they need to make in order to overcome their difficulties. This works on the time honored principle that the human brain tries to bring about what it focuses on (Q.7). This solution-focused approach can have a dramatic effect on motivating the individual to take the action they need to bring themselves out of their exhausted state. There is now some very strong evidence for the effectiveness of this brief form of therapy.[17]

In order to avoid or recover from depression, we also need to remember to meet our emotional needs (see Q.1), ensuring that we are giving ourselves the psychological "nutrition" to feel fulfilled in our lives. We may need to identify the resources we have (see Q.7) and develop our confidence and social skills in order to get "out and about" again (see Chapter 7). As we start to take up interesting activities again, mental or physical, serotonin levels in the brain increase, which regulate our REM sleep and make us feel further motivated to meet our needs and do the things we enjoy.

 If you think you are suffering from depression, you need to seek professional help (see Q.23).

CASE STUDY

Judith was forty-three years old and had a good relationship with her husband, two grown sons and a grandson, whom she loved looking after twice a week. She also ran a charity for women who suffer from domestic abuse. Generally she felt very content with her life and couldn't understand why she felt anxious so much of the time. Judith learned from a self-help book, about the effects of negative "black and white" thinking and how it can create anxiety by preventing the individual from seeing all the positive things in life and keeping them focused on all the "what if's."

Judith realized that she spent a large proportion of the day ruminating on thoughts such as, "What if my husband has an accident?" or "What if I can't raise the money to keep the charity going?" or "What if I become ill and can't look after my grandson?" All these thoughts were firing off the **fight-or-flight response** and because Judith tried to just divert herself away from these thoughts, without really looking at the evidence for or against them, she was left feeling highly anxious and out of control.

Judith began to tune into these thoughts and then write them down using 7/11 breathing (Q.4) to calm herself sufficiently to access her rational brain. She then began to write down evidence for and against each thought and then came up with more balanced ways of thinking. Having done this, every time she noticed herself thinking, "What if . . ." she pictured a big warning bell ringing in her head and recalled the more balanced thought she had come up with, using 7/11 breathing to keep her rational mind in charge. She also began to be more mindful of her language, again imagining ringing the bell in her head if she caught herself using "should's," "must's," and "ought's."

Within a few weeks Judith realized how she had almost started to laugh at herself when she starting "what if-ing." "What a waste of time that was!" she said to herself, if those thoughts popped up. She quickly began to feel more relaxed and more able to problem solve as challenges came up.

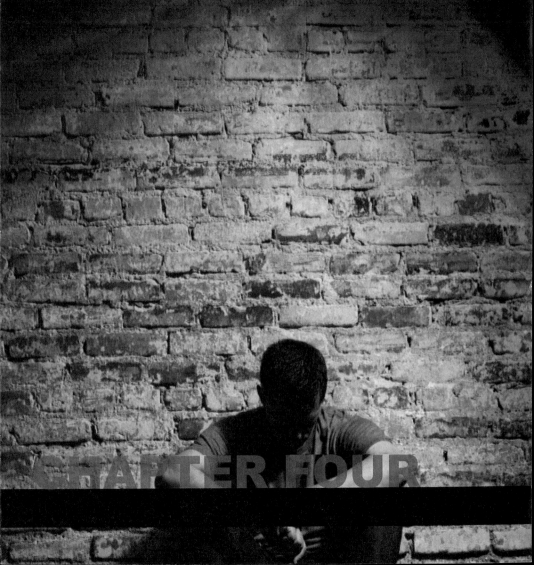

CHAPTER FOUR

Reducing Anger

Although we think of ourselves as fairly evolved creatures, the truth is when we get worked up, we very quickly get "emotionally high-jacked" and our intelligence plummets. This leaves us as a slave to our primitive brains, which were in control back in the days when we were cavemen.

Leading neurobiologist, Dan Siegel[18] calls this emotional high-jacking process "flipping your lid." He explains that, in very basic terms, we have two parts to our brain:

1. The old <u>primitive</u> part of our brain, the **limbic system**

   This controls basic survival instincts, hunger, sexual desire, and emotions.

   Because this part of our brain evolved at an early stage in human development, it is deep **inside** the brain.

2. The <u>intelligent</u> part of our brain, the cortex

   This part of our brain evolved at a later stage in our development. It is responsible for intelligent and rational thinking, including problem solving and strategic decision-making. It also performs the vital role of inhibiting and moderating the emotions and desires of the primitive "caveman brain." As civilized human beings, the cortex helps us to operate in a complex modern world without being a total slave to our more basic desires. The cortex, being the "newer part of the brain," covers the limbic system, **like a lid.**

When we are relatively calm, going about our day-to-day business, both parts of the brain work in harmony, moderating our emotions and behavior accordingly. However, when something really pushes our buttons, throwing us back in time to a past hurt or trauma, or touches a sensitive spot, the rational cortex becomes deactivated ("flips off") and we are left in the control of our emotionally charged, caveman brain, the limbic system. We literally "flip our lid!"

Anger robs us of clear thought, dignity and compassion. In this emotionally charged, unchecked state, we can say and do things that in our usual rational state, we wouldn't dream of! It is a dangerous place to be and can be the cause of relationship breakdown, job loss, property destruction and, at its worst, physical violence. Don't forget, we are in our most basic survival state at this time, often feeling that we are fighting for our lives, and with little intelligent thinking present to draw on.

Anger can also have a detrimental effect on our physical health. It draws blood to the head and away from our organs, making us more prone to heart disease and heart attack. In fact, anger is a stronger predictor of dying young from heart disease than high cholesterol or blood pressure.

26. How can I get my anger under control?

The good news is that there are several ways to quickly and effectively "flip our lid" back on when we feel ourselves becoming emotional.

1) Spot early warning signs

The starting point to getting back in control is to notice the process happening <u>early</u>. If you ignore the early warning signs and let the caveman brain take over, that's when you're in trouble and at a point of no return.

How do you know you are starting to "lose it?" Everyone has a physical reaction to the beginning of this process. Look at the diagram in Q.2 which shows the physical symptoms which may be present as part of the **fight-or-flight response** and which can kick in with heightened emotion like anger. Identify what your early warning signs are.

When you have identified what your body does to tell you that your lid is about to flip, don't let this sign go unchecked. For example, when your heart starts to pound, you need to act immediately. Try 7/11 breathing (Q.4) and then divert your attention to doing something to get your **adrenaline** levels down (see Q.12(1) for a list of emergency diversion strategies). Pick one and practice, practice, practice. This will help you to create a new response pathway for yourself, whereby as soon as you notice the fight-or-flight response triggering, you can take immediate action to stop it taking over. This will increase your sense of control and your mental well-being.

2) Tense and relax

If you are prone to quickly getting angry and you have been used to feeling tense or angry for a long time, you may find trying to use some of the relaxation tips and breathing techniques described in this book somewhat challenging. The following technique allows you to work with tension in the body and reduce it, by actually increasing it first. It is a good introduction to relaxation/breathing techniques for beginners and a very helpful way of beginning to experience how it feels to be relaxed and free from tension, especially when we have forgotten what that feels like.

This is not suitable for anyone who suffers with joint problems such as arthritis.

NOTE

Exercise 14. The tense and relax exercise

ON THE CD

3) The no. 1 emergency strategy

Expecting ourselves to stay in a situation which is highly provocative and remain calm and rational, is highly irrational. It just doesn't fit with how our brain works. Once the fight-or-flight response is triggered, our whole central nervous system is geared up to fight or run away from the situation (see Q.2). Trying to work against that instinct by staying in the situation and talking it out may only lead to disaster, as we have seen.

Our number one emergency strategy is to:

WALK AWAY!

When your buttons are pushed and you notice the physiological changes beginning to happen (as described in Q.2), give yourself some space as quickly as you can. Obviously if you are walking away from someone who may be further inflamed by your leaving, you need to briefly say that you are going in order to calm down and be able to talk properly. The other person needs to understand that you are not walking away because you don't think it's important, but really the opposite. Prepare a phrase that works for you, so that when you need to say it, it will come without you having to think too much (remember your thinking brain has shut down at this point!).

You could say something like:

"This is a really important issue and I want to talk properly about it, but I need to get a twenty minute time-out to calm down, then I will come back and discuss it with you."

Give yourself at least twenty minutes. If you go off for five minutes, although you will initially feel better, as soon as you are back in the situation your adrenaline levels will quickly rise again and you will be back to square one. In that twenty minutes, ideally take some exercise, for example, take a brisk walk, jog on the spot, run up and down the stairs or use 7/11 breathing (Q.4), all of which help you to calm down quickly. When you have calmed down, you could then use your thinking brain to put yourself in the other person's shoes. Ask yourself, "How would I feel in their situation?"

Anger, or indeed any intense, negative emotion, can be overwhelming. Even low levels can block rational thought, empathy and creative insight. In fact, it can lead us into a **trance** state, where we feel totally absorbed by it, and unable to see what is going on around us.

One way of breaking patterns of behavior which arise from anger and other emotions, is to tap into our natural ability to step back from ourselves and see the bigger picture. This means using our **observing self.** In this mode of awareness, we can put distance between the emotion and our actions and see that we are much more than the anger, rage, or jealousy. This helps us to understand how we may have become conditioned to react in certain ways, and to break the patterns which have unconsciously developed between our thoughts, emotions, and certain situations and people.

In order to engage the observing self, we need to learn how to calm ourselves, using 7/11 breathing (Q.4) or any of the relaxation techniques in Chapter 1. When we are relaxed, we can begin to move away from the kind of strong, negative self-talk going on in our heads which we have used to build and justify our feelings of anger.

Reflect on the following when you feel calm:

What are you saying to justify your anger, jealousy, etc.?
Would it stand up if put "on trial?"
What are your motivations to stop reacting in this emotional way?

Exercise 15. Observe and make changes

Through regular relaxation, we can also begin to see that there are other, more appropriate ways of meeting our emotional needs. Above all, when relaxation switches off the **fight-or-flight response** (Q.2), we can take a step back and observe ourselves acting more resourcefully in difficult situations, as Exercise 15 demonstrates.

Lynne was in her early sixties. All her children lived more than an hour away and so she didn't see them as much as she would like. She had been a housewife for many years but her husband was still working part-time. She felt resentful that her husband has chosen to continue to work as she felt that financially he didn't need to. Her husband also played golf twice a week and was active in charity work. Lynne found herself becoming aggressive and angry with her husband, particularly when she had been drinking alcohol. She would pick at things he said and often end up insulting him in a very personal way. This had resulted in situations such as loud arguments breaking out in restaurants, where Lynne would end up storming off in the middle of a meal. She also found that her children were becoming more distant from her because they feared her angry outbursts at family gatherings and didn't want to listen to her ranting about their father's "lack of consideration."

Lynne was beginning to feel overwhelmed by her anger and at times felt panicky and dizzy. She went to her physician who said she thought she might be depressed and Lynne agreed that might be true, although she didn't want to take antidepressants at this stage. Her doctor agreed to wait but gave her some Web site addresses with tips to help her manage her anger. Lynne worked with some of these ideas, and began to recognize the first sign that she was starting to feel angry. She realized that she first felt a tightening in her chest and some nausea. She started to employ the "tense and relax" exercise (Exercise 14 on the CD-ROM) as soon as she noticed that happening. She also spent some time doing the "Observe and make changes" exercise (Exercise 15 on the CD-ROM). This helped her to see that she had been behaving irrationally. She recognized that she needed to cut down on alcohol and decided to limit herself to one glass with a meal. She did seek some one-on-one therapy to help with letting go of some past traumas, as she could see now that was affecting her self-esteem and causing her to blame and criticize others, in particular, her husband.

Looking at her list of emotional needs (Q.1, Exercise 1), Lynne could see that she was scoring low on her need for achievement and being "stretched," as well as her sense of connection to the wider community. She found herself some voluntary work in a retirement community teaching pottery and also joined a book club. Within six weeks she noticed that she was feeling much more calm and positive within herself and toward others close to her.

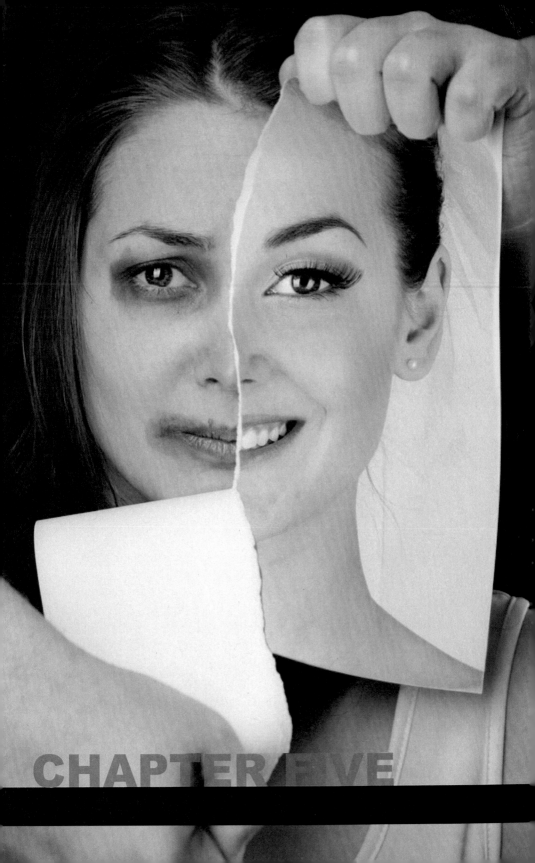

CHAPTER FIVE

Improving Physical Health and Sleep

28. Can the way I think affect my physical health?

The strong connection between our mind and our body is easily demonstrated by thinking about eating a lemon. Notice how quickly your mouth begins to pucker and fill with saliva, although there is no lemon there. Or how, when you remember a very embarrassing time, you might find yourself blushing, even though you are only thinking about the past. Dr Robert Ader was a founder of the field of psychoneuroimmunology (PNI) that has demonstrated communication pathways between our mind (thoughts, expectation, and the way we perceive life's events), our brain, hormones, immunity, and disease.[19] While worry, despair, and negative beliefs about our health or the treatment we are receiving can lead to poor health outcomes, for example, lowered immunity and slower wound healing, the reverse is equally valid. We can use the way we think and what we believe to enhance our health and immunity, whether for boosting our energy levels, recovering from injury or surgery, alleviating the symptoms of particular conditions, reducing the side effects from medication (Q.32), increasing the number and activity of disease-fighting T cells, or lowering levels of stress hormones and blood pressure.

When we want to improve our health or energy, we can create a powerful visualization of ourselves as full of wellness, following the guidelines for visualization in Q.6. What do we look like? How do we move? What do we sound like when we speak? For example, we might imagine ourselves with a smiling face, feel ourselves moving with vigor, saying a bright "Good morning" to people we meet. As we relax into our imagined state of wellness, the body will react as if we are experiencing these sensations for real (just as we produced saliva at the thought of that lemon). We might also visualize life after recovery from injury, illness or surgery, doing all those things we look forward to doing. Again, we can see ourselves full of life and good energy, notice what it feels like when we swim, or run, or return to our hobbies, or play with our grandchildren.

We know that exercise is good for our health as it stimulates the production of "feel good" brain chemicals, called endorphins, in our bodies, and also provides an outlet for high circulating levels of stress hormones caused by anxiety. Even while we may not be able to exercise, visualizing doing it will stimulate the same neural connections and bring benefits to our physical well-being. If you find this difficult to do, remember a time when you were physically active. What did it feel like? "Bathe" yourself in those memories and sensations.

Our emotional response to illness can have a crucial bearing on our recovery and future health.[20] When we are unwell, it is important to separate the illness from our core identity. Talking about "my migraine," "my arthritis," "my cancer" or "my heart disease" allows our condition to define who we are. In addition, focusing on our symptoms helps to maintain them. Instead, we can ensure that we continue to take control over the smaller things in our life and meet our human needs for fulfillment (Q.1).

 PRACTICAL TIP Take some time to relax. In your mind, consider the following statement: "When I think of myself as full of wellness and strength, I am like a . . ." Allow an image to emerge. An example might be a strong tree, deeply rooted in the earth but spreading and reaching upward into the sky. You might base your image on an interest you have, for example, as a surfer, riding a huge, shining wave. Keep returning to your image whenever you are relaxing, adding more detail as it emerges. You can then begin to access it when you are feeling anxious or worried, tired or down, or when you are about to go into a challenging situation. Notice the positive effect it has on your mind and body.

29. Is stress linked to illness?

Stress adversely affects both our behavior and our physical health. Stress and anxiety may prompt us into a host of unhealthy behaviors, for example, smoking, taking harmful drugs, eating the wrong foods, indulging in sexually risky behavior, avoiding exercise, driving too fast, and so on. Many health problems have psychological elements and may be exacerbated by stress or even triggered by stress, including skin conditions, allergies, digestive complaints, high blood pressure, migraine, cardiac illness, and auto-immune diseases like cancer and ME. When we are anxious or worried we trigger the **fight-or-flight response** (Q.2) and the body produces stress hormones. What evolved to save our lives in real danger, may now make us ill. As the stress hormones remain in our system long-term, many of our normal, health-giving functions are suppressed and this can lead to a host of physical and mental problems, including raised blood pressure, shallow breathing, lowered energy and sex drive, suppressed immune response, poor digestion and disrupted sleep, and "fuzzy" thinking.

Finding ways of reducing stress in our lives prevents this vicious cycle occurring. This book contains many ways of avoiding and lowering stress, starting with some of the basics included in Chapters 1 and 2, and moving on to challenging negative thinking (Chapter 3), reducing anger (Chapter 4) and setting achievable goals for doing the things you enjoy (Chapter 6).

30. How can I use my mind to promote good physical health and healing?

When we experience physical health problems, we can learn to harness the power of the mind to "self-soothe," where we deeply relax and allow our minds to create healing **metaphors** for our well-being, illness, symptoms, or discomfort. We all use metaphors to describe our physical condition. For example, we may talk about pain using words like "burning," "stabbing," "dull," or "nagging." We can utilize these same metaphors as a key to creating new ones which are self-soothing and healing. We could imagine a cool liquid bathing an affected part of our body to soothe away "burning" sensations, or a colored light flowing into an area of "dull" discomfort. The metaphor engages the imaginative right hemisphere of the brain and bypasses the conscious, rational part of our mind which may be negative or resistant. In this way, it "speaks" to the unconscious, where we can try out a new way of seeing the world and new patterns of responding. This process has been utilized by hypnotherapists with excellent results in reducing symptoms in certain conditions which are difficult to treat, such as irritable bowel syndrome.[21]

We can elaborate our metaphors into healing stories, for example, imagining our immune system as a castle that needs defending and the guards doing their job well, or our high blood pressure as a narrow river which needs unblocking from weeds, rocks and silt, so that it can widen and flow more quietly and smoothly. Milton Erickson, the American psychiatrist who pioneered innovative approaches to clinical **hypnotherapy**, was a great story teller and used stories to **reframe** his patients' experiences of illness and pain.[22]

PRACTICAL TIP

Identify some of the metaphors you use to describe your physical condition, symptoms, or discomfort, including words, shapes, colors, sounds, etc. Then move on to the activity on the accompanying CD-ROM.

Self-soothing can also help us to think more calmly and rationally about the health-related decisions we take in our lives and the choices we make about our lifestyles.

ON THE CD

Exercise 16. Create a soothing space

31. Can I use my mind to reduce pain?

All pain has a psychological element. We know that pain and other distressing bodily sensations, for example, tinnitus or skin irritation, can seem much worse when we focus on them, or when we are anxious, stressed, or depressed. In fact, pain seems to put us into a **trance**, narrowing our focus of attention so that the experience is heightened and all-consuming. This makes it difficult to consciously divert away to more pleasant things.

The "gate control" theory of pain[23] suggests that pain signals compete with other signals as they reach the spinal cord and can be switched on or off depending on the priority of other messages. A well-known example is our natural impulse to shout or jump up and down when we stub a toe, rather than just stand still and focus on the pain. Pain that accompanies safe and pleasant experiences may be classified as irrelevant and never reach the brain. This suggests that getting absorbed in what we enjoy can help to block our awareness of pain.

When you are experiencing pain or discomfort, grade its intensity from 0 percent (not present at all) to 100 percent (as bad as you could possibly imagine). Grading or **scaling** pain in this way engages the thinking mind, distracting away from the emotional overwhelm of the experience. It also enables you to notice finer distinctions and improvements from day to day.

When someone is in pain, the emotional brain is activated and as we saw in Chapters 3 and 4, they may be prone to inflexible, "black and white," "all or nothing," thinking in relation to their experience. Many of the techniques introduced in Chapter 3 for breaking down or challenging this style of thinking may be helpful.

Learning to stay relaxed is the first step to diminishing the hold painful or unpleasant sensations can have on our consciousness (see Q.6). We can then begin to focus on pleasant events and sensations to distract us away from pain. Laughter is a wonderful, natural medicine for pain, increasing levels of serotonin (the "happy chemical") in the brain, and diminishing anxiety and stress related to the experience of pain.

The mind has the ability to change or reduce physical sensation. The American psychiatrist and clinical hypnotherapist, Milton Erickson, clearly demonstrated the importance of suggestion and expectation in the experience of pain (Q.22). As a result of his work and those of hypnotherapists working in the field of pain, we know that we can learn to alter pain into less disturbing sensations like tingling or warmth, using self-soothing **metaphors** (Q.30), or use our minds to "turn down" the pain. This helps to give us back a sense of control, which is important in avoiding anxiety, negative thinking, and depression.

When we feel disassociated from something, we feel less emotional about it. You can distance yourself from pain by imagining you are far away from it, in another room, or another place, or even "outside of yourself" and thereby free of pain. This can be helpful for long-term, chronic pain.

Exercise 17. Turn down that pain

Always see a doctor about any pain you are experiencing before undertaking any pain relief activity.

32. How can I use my mind to get the most benefit from medical treatment?

The **placebo** effect is a well-researched phenomenon, showing that positive expectations by both patient and healthcare provider can positively affect health outcomes. Our minds are enormously susceptible to suggestion and the power of our beliefs. When we believe that a particular treatment will be beneficial, or when a physician seems confident and concerned, our bodies are more likely to respond favorably, even in the case of "sugar pills" which contain no active substances. In fact, sugar pills have been found to cause profound changes in the same area of the brain as the drugs they are masquerading as. The active ingredient seems to be the *power of belief* that the patients have received a powerful and effective treatment. For example, research has shown that a placebo given by injection is more effective than if given by a tablet, because the injection is seen as stronger medicine.[24]

In the same way positive expectations can enhance the effects of our treatment, patients who expect the worst health-wise, tend to get just that. Factors which feed our negative expectations can lead to a negative or nocebo effect. Examples include believing that you are prone to a particular disease, being told by the physician that you will experience particular side-effects from a drug or that a procedure will hurt, or noticing a look of doubt on the doctor's face when she is talking about the low risk of a given procedure. At its very worst, there are many anecdotal reports of patients being told they have three to six months to live and dying "dutifully" on the final day of their "prescribed" time span.

Cultivate feelings of gratitude toward your healthcare givers, your medicine or the surgical procedure you are about to have. Feelings of deep gratitude create positive expectations and prime our bodies to respond to the benefits of what is being offered.

PRACTICAL TIP

Exercise 18. The inner smile

ON THE CD

33. How can I improve my sleep patterns?

Sleep is an entirely natural process, one that we didn't even have to think about when we were babies or children. However, our busy adult lives can raise our levels of stress to an extent where we start to worry about sleep. At night our continued thinking can stimulate our waking minds into mental activity, whether problem solving, list-making, or anxious imaginings. In fact, many of us do all sorts of things to "try" to get to sleep, rather than getting our conscious minds "out of the way" so that we can allow sleep to take over.

Many of the difficulties we regularly experience in living, including difficulty in sleeping, arise from the patterns of thinking and behaviors we have learned, however unintentionally and consciously. For example, we may regularly postpone going to bed because we are channel-hopping on the TV or playing computer games. If sleep has become a problem, we may think about going upstairs or getting ready for bed with anxiety or even dread. Using a "sleep hygiene" approach can start to change unhelpful patterns and stimulate thinking and activities which pave the way for a good night's sleep.

"Sleepy mind" checklist:
- Avoid stimulating activities an hour before bedtime, such as watching TV, playing computer games, or surfing the Internet.
- Minimize persistent worrying by keeping a notebook of worry "topics" which you can write in at any time (see also Q.10).
- Try to instill a routine around bedtime and getting-up time.
- If you wake in the night, avoid turning the light on or looking at the time. Focus on your breath coming and going from the belly area or on relaxing the body, starting from the feet and working up to the head.
- If you don't get back to sleep within about thirty minutes, get up and sit in a cool, dark room. If you must do something, make sure it is a boring, non-stimulating activity, rather than something you enjoy. As soon as you are really tired, leave the task and return to bed. Focus on your breathing or body relaxation again.
- If you are still awake after another twenty to thirty minutes, get up and do another boring task or pick up on the one you left. Once your mind realizes that it will be punished for not sleeping (rather than rewarded), it will learn to get you off to sleep at night.

You also may need to look at physical factors which might be affecting your sleep, like alcohol, caffeine, timing of meals and exercise, body heat and hormonal imbalance.

Make your bedroom a place you associate with sleep. If possible, remove the TV, computer, office, or studying area to another room. Control lighting and noise by using an eye mask or ear plugs if necessary. You can also interrupt the usual bedtime patterns and associations by doing your bedtime reading, sleeping, or washing in a different place, or rearranging your bedroom.

The **CBT** approach looks at thoughts, actions, and feelings and can help to change unhelpful responses toward going to bed. Try the next exercise on the CD-ROM.

Exercise 19. Changing sleep patterns

If sleep is a persistent problem, see your GP to rule out underlying health problems, and for assessment and advice.

34. How can I get off to sleep?

Sleeping is not about "switching off" the brain, but rather, activating it in a different way. When we have difficulty in sleeping, it is often because we are disturbed by the external sounds and sensations and try to block them out. However, we can use the sounds and other features around us to encourage the natural "auto-symbolic affect." This occurs as our attention begins to turn inward and sensory input from the outside starts getting altered into fragments of dreams. For example, the sound of a dripping tap might

The more practiced you become at relaxing, the more easily you will drift into sleep and the deeper your sleep will be. Use the relaxation techniques in Q.6 to take a short, deep rest during the day. This will boost your energy for the rest of the day and prepare the ground for getting off to sleep at night.

symbolically become a running stream, or the warmth of the bedclothes might become the feel of sunshine on a beach. These visualizations help us to drift into trance or sleep.

ON THE CD

Exercise 20. Three things to take you into sleep

CASE STUDY

Beverley was thirty-five and was being treated for breast cancer. She knew that staying calm and positive would have many benefits, physically, mentally, and emotionally, so she began to practice deep relaxation every day. During her treatment, she visualized a colored light washing through her body, dissolving cancer cells, strengthening her immune cells, and repairing her body following surgery. She saw herself receiving the very best treatment, staying relaxed and at ease, with all the support she needed around her. She noticed that she felt gradually less fearful and more in control of how she responded to the challenges of her illness. She started to find contentment in small, everyday pleasures, such as a sunny day, a visit from a friend, or some unexpected kindness from her healthcare givers. This helped her to stay patient with her treatment and herself, taking each day as it came.

As a keen horse rider, Beverley developed her own inner mental **metaphor** for strength and resilience, based on galloping along a beautiful beach on a black stallion. She imagined what it would feel like to ride so fast and freely, feeling the wind in her hair, smelling and tasting the saltiness of the ocean, and hearing the horse's hooves pounding along the damp sand. She pictured merging with the power of the horse, strong and resilient. She found that this practice helped her to stay hopeful and boosted her energy.

As her treatment came to an end, Beverley began to visualize a time when she had felt full of energy and well-being in the past, really focusing on the physical sensations in her body and the thoughts associated with this time. She then imagined herself in the future, with the same feelings and thoughts, vibrant and healthy, doing all the things she loved to do. She noticed how this helped her to put her cancer treatment behind her and focus on her progress toward being fully well again.

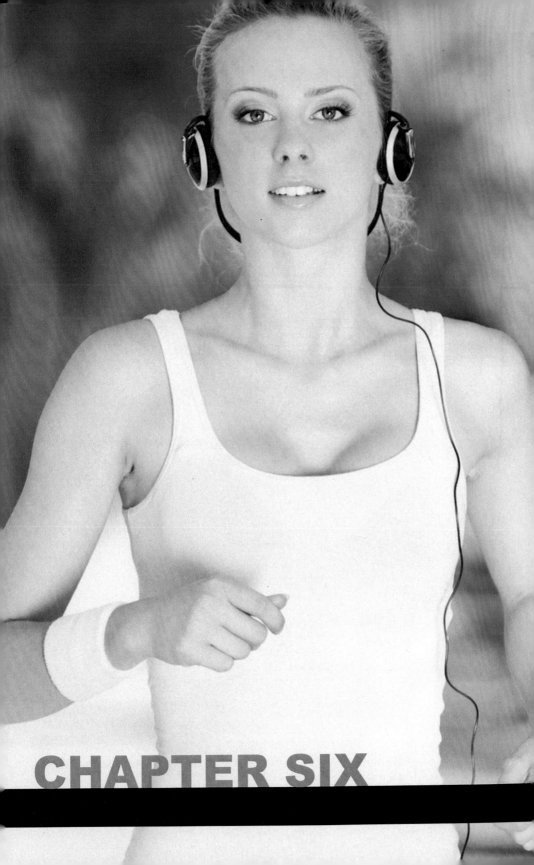

CHAPTER SIX

Set Goals and Boost Motivation

35. How can setting and achieving goals improve my sense of well-being?

It is so easy to get caught up in the busyness of day-to-day life, that sometimes we can lose sight of the bigger picture and what our most important goals are. Taking time to set goals can draw you back to your core beliefs and values and help you bring things into your life that really matter. It can also help you to let go of what's using up your time and energy without being of any real value to you. Learning how to set realistic goals that you can achieve gives you a sense of control, motivating you to find ways of feeling fulfilled and more content in life.

Writing your own "eulogy" can help you refocus on what is really important to you.

PRACTICAL TIP

Imagine your headstone. If your family, friends, and colleagues were asked to write on it what they thought about you when you were living, what would you want them to write?

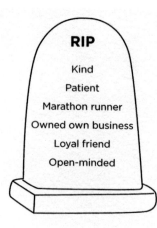

RIP

Kind

Patient

Marathon runner

Owned own business

Loyal friend

Open-minded

◄ FIGURE 6.1 My eulogy

If it commemorated your proudest achievements, what would you want these to be?

The next activity takes this exercise a stage further, helping you to begin to set some goals in your life.

Exercise 21. Goals from the grave

36. How can I begin to prioritize the goals I have?

The number one biggest mistake we can make when trying to bring positive change into our lives is to make our goals too big, or to set too many of them, so that we inevitably feel overwhelmed and then don't do anything.

It is helpful to use goal setting techniques that can help you to prioritize and break down your goals so that you have a clear beginning and end point, rather than getting lost in the process and giving up. One such technique uses the **NLP** concept of "chunking down," moving from the general to the specific. In this case, you can try breaking a big goal into smaller, more precise "chunks" so that it becomes manageable and achievable. The following exercise uses this chunking down approach.

Exercise 22. Get it all down on paper

37. How can I become more successful at achieving my goals?

There is an art to setting and achieving goals. Approaching it in a haphazard way seldom works. If this was not true, we would all be slimmer, fitter, have given up drinking/smoking, taken up new hobbies, and started that business. How many break room conversations start, "I really must . . ."?

Generally speaking, if you structure your goals, you have far more chance of achieving them. This then increases your energy to continue setting more goals and life moves on in the way you <u>really</u> want it to. Contrast this to just being swept along and reacting to what life throws at us. It is true to say that when we feel in control of our lives, we are at our happiest. Setting and achieving goals gives us a great sense of being in control. We get a sense of moving forward and achieving things, rather than a sense of staying stuck, which can make life dull and uninteresting.

One way of ensuring goals are achievable is to "smarten" them up. Using the "SMART" approach can shape your goals and hugely increase your chance of achieving them.

SMART

S = Specific: Make sure you narrow down what it is you want to achieve.

M = Measurable: How will you know when you have achieved what it is you have set out to achieve?

A = Attainable: Make sure the goal is something within your reach, not something you have to wait for or don't have the resources at present to realize.

R = Realistic: Don't make the goal too difficult. If anything, make it too easy, then when you achieve it, you have an increased sense of your abilities and more confidence to set and achieve more complex goals.

T = Time related: Put a timeframe on your goal of when you will achieve it, rather than leaving it open ended. This will give you a deadline to work to, so that you don't just leave it and think you will get around to it at some point.

So, here is an example:

You need to get fit; you've tried the gym and hated it. You used to enjoy badminton but don't have anyone to play with. Instead of waiting for a partner to drop in your lap, you decide it's time to take action and find one.

Specific: To find a partner to play with once a week for an hour, at either of the two closest venues to me.

Measurable: I will have achieved it when I am playing badminton once a week.

Attainable: I will put notices up at those two venues, as I know I can get to either one easily. I will also call both of them to see if they have any lessons or leagues I can join.

Realistic: I will play just once a week as I know I can manage that.

Time related: I will drop the notices in on Saturday morning and I will call both clubs by the end of this week.

You are now well on your way to increasing your fitness!

Remember, that at first you might need to write goals down in this structured way but soon, as with learning any new skills, the process will start to feel more natural and you will find that you can achieve more and more.

Exercise 23. Smarten up your goals

38. What's the best technique for motivating myself when I feel "stuck"?

Are there any New Year's resolutions you haven't got around to yet? Why is it that, although we have all the very best intentions of making positive changes in our lives, ones that will be of enormous benefit, somehow these changes just never seem to happen?

One big unknown around setting and achieving goals is this:

When there is will and emotion in conflict, emotion always wins![25]

Here's an example of how this works in day-to-day life. You know you really need to start doing some exercise. Your doctor has told you that your weight is really becoming a problem (you're officially "obese!"); your spouse has started tennis again and you feel guilty about that. When you do walk uphill, you notice your breathing becomes labored and you feel a bit dizzy. However, when you get home from work each night and it's cold and dark, you sit on the sofa feeling cozy and relaxed and the thought of getting up and out to the gym is very unattractive. You then decide that you'll just stay in tonight but definitely go tomorrow. You know that you <u>should</u> go tonight (will) but you just don't <u>feel</u> like it (emotion)

So, this is where we get stuck! The trick is to stop waiting to <u>feel</u> like doing it and to accept that this is just not going to happen. Every top athlete will tell you that often the way they get themselves out to train is by forcing themselves to do it. This doesn't sound very appealing, but here's a trick that will really help:

Overcome "stuck-ness" by following the "five minute rule." When you have a task which you know you need to do but just don't feel like doing, make it easy on yourself. Recognizing that your will and emotions will be in conflict, make a deal with yourself that you will only do the task for five minutes. Suddenly, it seems a lot less daunting, it's only five minutes after all!

In all likelihood, once you have done five minutes, you will have bypassed your resistance and be in **flow** with the activity so that you want to carry on (see Q.50). However, just in case you don't, you have still achieved five minutes of the activity, which is better than doing nothing and is a step in the right direction.

CASE STUDY

Andrew is twenty-two and has suffered with social anxiety for as long as he can remember. He often felt "on the edge of things" at school and with groups of friends. At work, he feels things are easier as he has a role and purpose, but when he is socializing he often feels people think he is quiet and boring. When Andrew thinks about his eulogy he realizes that others might feel he is "unfriendly" as he often withdraws from people. He really wants to come across as more "friendly" and "open." He decides that he could take the first step by asking his squash partner, Matt, if he would like a drink after their game when they play next Tuesday. He knows that this might be short notice, so he decides that if Matt says he can't make it, he will ask him to do it next week.

He plans that when they have a drink he will have three questions to ask Matt: "How is his work going? Is he planning a vacation?" And, "Does he play other sports other than squash?" He also decides he will tell Matt about his plans to move to a new house and the film he watched last night. He also vows to make a real effort to smile and remain sitting upright with his arms unfolded, as he has learned this will make him look and feel more relaxed. Armed with these specific goals, topics, and questions for discussion, he feels much less nervous about inviting his friend for a drink.

Health, Happiness, Success.

Self Esteem

Self
Confidence

Emotional
Intelligence

CHAPTER SEVEN

Enhancing Assertiveness, Self-Esteem, and Confidence

Generally in life, our self-esteem will ebb and flow. Sometimes we can feel we have so little control over this that somehow these fluctuations "just happen." However, this is rarely the case! When our self-esteem dips, it may well be that someone said something, or that something happened which triggered a memory or pattern from the past. These memories or patterns are often stored unconsciously, that is to say, they are not at the forefront of our minds. This means that we may not even be aware of them being triggered by a current event, we just have a sense of feeling okay, then not feeling okay. Our baseline of how we generally feel about ourselves does stem largely from the early messages we receive in life. If you know that these were very negative over a long period of time, you may benefit from one-on-one therapy to help let go of them and move on with your life.

However, there is one key skill to boosting our self-esteem and keeping it at a generally higher level, so that when things come along that may have previously floored us, we can keep our head above water and still feel okay. This skill is linked to our emotional need of having a sense of achievement. We all need to ensure that we have a range of activities in our lives which we find stimulating, and which gives us a sense of satisfaction when we complete them. This really can be anything from playing a musical instrument, supporting a friend in a time of trouble, having a satisfying job, or being able to arrange a vase of flowers beautifully. It

Exercise 24. Take practical steps to better self-esteem

really doesn't matter what it is, but there is truth in the saying, *"We are what we do!"*

40. What techniques can I use day to day to feel more confident?

One of the most commonly reported psychological complaints is feeling a lack of confidence. Janice Davies, who specializes in the study of self-confidence and is known as "The Attitude Specialist," has found that 95 percent of children and adults report feeling a lack of confidence at some point in their lives.[26] Richard Lovelace, a psychotherapist, found that low confidence and self-esteem is closely linked to how we deal with stress,[27] in that if we are suffering from low self-esteem, we will also find life's challenges harder to deal with. It is, of course, the case that some people have had a start in life which has made them feel fundamentally secure and confident. However, it is surprising how many of us who present as very confident, often feel shy and nervous on the inside.

While confidence levels can be significantly affected by our early parenting and the messages we received as small children about our worth, it is also true to say that they are not set in stone. There is plenty we can do as adults to dramatically increase our self-confidence.

We have already seen that an important factor in maintaining self-esteem comes from engaging in activities which we can gain a sense of achievement from. One additional, powerful technique for developing confidence is based on the old saying, *"Fake it 'til you make it!"* As long ago as 1894, the philosopher, William James, pronounced that, "If you want a quality, act as if you already have it." Plenty of research since has shown that acting as though you feel a particular way—including confident—leads to really feeling that way.[28] The following activity, based on this premise, is particularly

Exercise 25. Borrow someone else's confidence!

ON THE CD

helpful when you know you have an event coming up which you feel nervous about and know you need a confidence boost.

41. How can I say "No!"?

Research shows that happy people know how to set their boundaries. One UK-based workplace study in 2001 showed that being assertive and "disagreeable" is even linked to earning more money![29] Trying to please all the people all of the time has a negative pay-off—you lose out. If you are a caring and considerate person, you can easily fall in the trap of saying yes to everyone and everything, just because you don't want to seem "bad" or "selfish."

The problem with this scenario is that sooner or later your self-esteem plummets! Think about it, if you are always putting others' needs before your own, the message you are giving to yourself is something like, "I am bottom of the pile, everyone else comes before me, I don't matter."

Of course, doing something helpful or kind for another person can be rewarding and also valuable in terms of meeting our need for emotional connection with others (Q.1), but it is all a case of balance.

When someone requests something of you, (whether it doesn't seem essential, or you know deep down that it might actually be good for you) if your instant internal response is negative, listen to it. For example, you might get that niggling feeling in your stomach or a tightening in the chest. This is your intuition telling you this isn't going to work for you. So, just say "No!"

It is really important to use the word "No," rather than skirting around it or making up "fluffy" excuses. Avoiding the word might feel easier because it is less like a rejection. However, this is less helpful for the other person, because they are left not knowing quite where they stand. Remember that you don't have to give an excuse or convoluted explanation; you have the <u>right</u> to say "No." You might simply say, "No, that's not possible. I appreciate you need help with this but I am just not able to help at this time," or, "No, I'm not able to help you with that."

The best way to start this new habit is with really small requests, so that you get practice in fairly low risk situations. Remember to use the word "No" wherever possible, because it gives a clear message to the requester and may result in less attempts at persuasion. For instance, when a telemarketer phones, you could say right at the start of the call, "No, I am not interested in talking to you about this subject, goodbye." You might purposefully get near a charity seller in the street, then when they approach, you can say, "No, thank you."

Spend some time thinking of other situations where you can practice using the word "No" without feeling compelled to make up excuses, so that when a request comes that you really need to turn down, it will feel much easier to do so. Always remember that you are only rejecting a request, not the person making the request. You may find that people are initially a little shocked or even angry with you when you say "No," especially if they are used to getting their own way with you! But if they are true friends, they will recover quickly and over time, have much more respect for you. This will, in turn, increase your self-esteem!

42. How can I use my body language to enhance the effectiveness of my communications?

When you are trying to get your point across and you notice that people just aren't listening, or you repeatedly find that people talk over you or just don't hear what you are saying, it might not be <u>what</u> you are saying, but the <u>way</u> you are saying it.

The importance of "non-verbal communication" (that is, what you are communicating via your posture, gestures, facial expressions and tone, volume and pace of your voice) is recognized by social psychologists as being extremely important. Some say that it accounts for as much as 70 percent of the impact of your communication, leaving only 30 percent for your words to have any influence![30] Although this is a debatable statistic, because precise measurement is difficult, the relative importance of non-verbal communication is certainly worth paying attention to.

 Watch films of people who you perceive as confident and borrow the qualities of their non-verbal communication.

It is very common, when you are feeling under pressure to get a communication "right" in tricky circumstances, to over-focus on <u>what</u> we say, rather than <u>how</u> we deliver it.

 Exercise 26. Make non-verbal communication work for you

43. How can I continue to assert my needs, when others are very persuasive or powerful?

When we are under pressure from others or we are at a low ebb within ourselves, we can feel that we have to give an instant response to a request asked of us. But this is only a rule that we have made up for ourselves. If you are someone who struggles to draw a line, and often ends up doing things you really don't want to be doing, learning to set and stick to boundaries could really help. A well-known assertiveness technique is to <u>delay your response</u>, so that you won't get caught off guard and agree to something you might not want to do. By delaying your response, you give yourself time to think and consider:

1. Is this actually a reasonable request?

2. Is it something I am able to do without feeling over-burdened?

3. Is it something I <u>want</u> to do?

When you have considered these questions, in your own time, then you will be able to give an honest, meaningful answer, rather than agreeing on the hoof and regretting it later.

Reclaim some power by <u>delaying your response</u>. Be armed with a phrase that gives you space to think. Then, when someone requests something of you which you feel in your gut might not be a good thing to agree to, you can simply say something like:

"I need to think about that and get back to you."

The person will probably want to know roughly when that might be, so if it's possible, give them a time or day when you will let them know your response. If you feel you are not able to give them a specific time, you can just say that you will let them know "as soon as possible."

Remember, if your gut is saying "No," then by going against that instinct and saying "Yes," you are chipping away at your own self-esteem. You are giving yourself the message that your needs are not important and, consequently, that <u>you</u> are not important. This is a slippery slope toward feeling depressed.

Exercise 27. Be like a broken record!

ON THE CD

Being assertive means being equal to others, that is, being respectful of others <u>and</u> yourself; you both deserve that!

CASE STUDY

Emma was twenty-eight and had recently moved to a new town to be with her boyfriend. She left a job that she loved and was very successful at, in order to move down. She did have friends in the new town as she had lived there as a child. She got a new job in a different field that she wasn't so familiar with. A few months after the move, she started to feel very low and was experiencing more and more self-doubt.

Emma went to see an old friend for the weekend and started talking to the friend about how she was feeling. The friend helped her to realize that she had lost her sense of achievement in work as she was not feeling like she was doing it well and was not getting feedback from her new boss. Emma also saw that her old friends in the new town really had different interests to her and she often felt uninteresting in their company.

Emma decided she had to talk to her boss about changing aspects of her job and also asking for feedback. She e-mailed her boss and asked for a meeting. After that weekend, she then began preparing for the meeting, by working out what aspects of her job she felt she did well and aspects of her job she needed more support with. The night before the meeting she prepared by taking some time out and using the "Step down" exercise (see Exercise 3 and Track 3). When she was relaxed she began to visualize her friend Mia at work, (whom she admired for her laid-back confidence) and "borrowed" her posture, smile, and way of saying what she would like to be different. She then visualized herself talking to her boss with those qualities. She kept running this film in her mind and then added a breezy soundtrack to it!

Just before the meeting, Emma practiced the countdown exercise again and visualized herself walking in with an upright posture, smiling and being clear about what she wanted to be different. In the meeting, Emma was pleasantly surprised that her boss did agree to some of her requests, and following this, she did start to feel better at work. She also decided to join a running club as she knew she needed to meet more people with common interests.

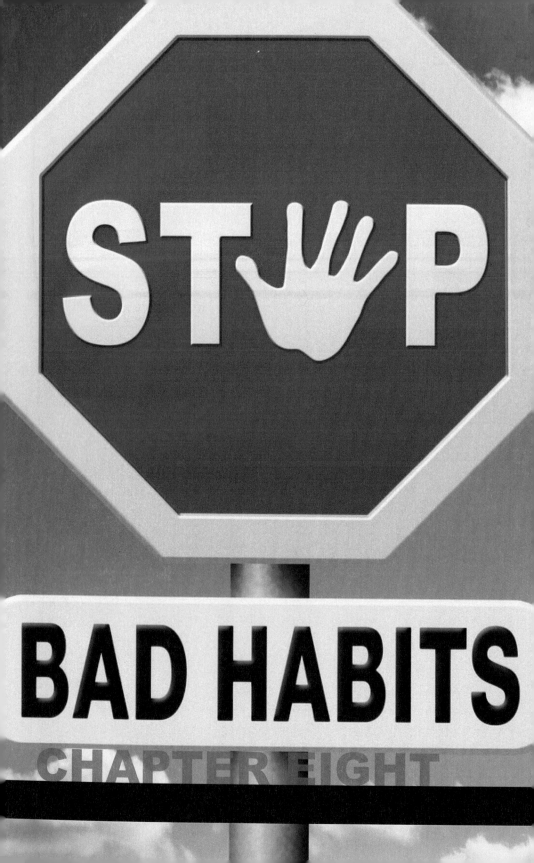

Changing Unhelpful Habits and Patterns

The way the brain has evolved over millions of years is a mind-boggling process. As a species, it has taken us from monkeys to intelligent beings, able to juggle huge amounts of information, and function in an increasingly complicated economic, political, and social world.

There are certain mechanisms within the brain that drive this process, enabling us to grow physically, emotionally, and intellectually, and giving us the incentive to continue developing, to try new things and to keep "upping our game." When we use our brains in an evolutionary way, this mechanism works perfectly for us, enabling us to live life to the fullest and to fulfill our human needs (Q.1). However, when we are overwhelmed with stress, for whatever reason, this mechanism can work against us, leading us into addictive patterns of behavior. This is when we begin to rely more and more on "chemical hits" within the brain to feel okay.

This potentially addictive process involves **dopamine**, which is a chemical that is released into our bloodstream in order to get us to take action. So, an example of this process working well, would be as follows:

> You take up canoeing. The first week, you really struggle co-ordinating everything you need to, you fall out several times and feel a bit stupid, but there is a friendly bunch of people around and you have fun. During the week, you start to feel excited about the next week's lessons, you expect to enjoy them and you look forward to it. The next week comes and you get a bit better with the technical side of things, staying in

the canoe for longer. You get a sense of achievement and start to get "the bug" for it, increasingly looking forward to future lessons, always expecting to have fun. This process of expecting fun, having fun, getting better at something, then wanting more, is dopamine working at its best for us. Dopamine is released every time we have a positive expectation; it drives us forward to complete that expectation by taking action. You can see how this enables us to evolve by getting our emotional needs met—feeling fulfilled and realizing dreams and expectations of the future.

However, when we are overwhelmed by emotion and stress and our focus is narrowed and bleak, our expectations of the future are not always positive. This is when we may look for "instant hits" to pick us up, fill a hole or just escape for what feels too painful to look at. So, in this situation, the role of dopamine can be misused by the brain and can lead us into serious trouble. Here's an example of how this might happen:

Work is very stressful and your relationship is going through a difficult patch. You have always enjoyed a glass of wine with dinner but recently have started having a couple before dinner too. During the stress of the day, you start to fantasize about that first glass of wine, how cool and crisp it will be, the first hit of alcohol relaxing your muscles as you sink down in your favorite chair, with the day behind you. You are creating an expectation of how wonderful that experience will be. When you get home, you have been thinking about how lovely that first sip will be for so long, you can't wait, and given what a day it has been, you feel you deserve it, so you bypass your soft drink and go straight for the wine. It is nice, but doesn't quite give you the pleasure you expected, so you have another. In no time at all, you've drank over half the bottle. You decide to cancel plans with friends as you can't drive now and you are just not in the mood. This further impacts on the difficulties you are having with your partner.

In both these situations, you build tolerance to the source of pleasure. This works well when you are pursuing a healthy pleasure that stretches you (as in the canoeing example) because it enables you to work at getting better and better, because you want more and more challenge. As you improve, you get more and more natural chemical hits from endorphins ("feel-good" hormones in your body) and feel happier and more alive. But in the wine drinking example, the process becomes destructive. As you build up tolerance, you need more and more alcohol to get that "hit," leading to physical health problems and a more isolated, miserable life where your emotional needs are increasingly neglected. This makes you vulnerable to depression, anxiety, and other serious problems.

 PRACTICAL TIP Are you aware of any destructive patterns of behavior in your life? Be honest with yourself by reflecting on whether there are things that take up your time and energy and draw you away from more meaningful, stretching activities. Be on your guard, these activities are the ones that can easily get out of control, if you allow your brain to <u>trick</u> you into thinking they will make you happy.

Use the techniques in this chapter to get these behaviors under control and allow your intelligent brain to get back in the driver's seat of life's journey!

45. Why do I keep failing at giving up unwanted habits?

Prochaska and DiClemente developed a model called "The cycle of change" in 1984, when they were studying how smokers were able to give up their habit.[31] The cycle describes the psychological process of giving up a habit, whatever that habit might be. What is so useful to understand from this model is that breaking addictive habits is generally not a linear process. It is often a case that "slipping up" or "relapse" is actually part of a process of stopping completely. A recent study at Coventry University in the UK showed that the average number of times a long-term smoker gives up is seven times.[32]

The worst enemy of breaking habits is not relapse; it is self-sabotage! The bully of addiction says something like, *"Oh well, you have had one cigarette/alcoholic drink/food binge/cut, and now you've failed, so you may as well do the job properly and have another,"* or, *"You've failed again, you will never kick this habit, you are not like other people so don't try to pretend you are."* This is where the real trouble starts, not with the relapse itself.

The cycle of change shows us that relapse is completely normal and that in fact, we learn something new every time we relapse. Have a look at the model:

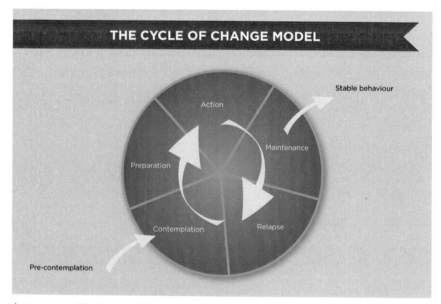

▲ FIGURE 8.1 The Cycle of Change model

The stages of change are as follows:

Pre-contemplation (not ready): Not yet acknowledging that there is a problem behavior that needs to be changed

Contemplation: Acknowledging that there is a problem, weighing up the pro's and con's of change, but not yet ready or sure of wanting to make a change

Action: Changing behavior/stopping the habit

Maintenance: Maintaining the behavior change

Relapse: Having a "slip up"

Sometimes, after a relapse we end up going around the whole cycle again. For example, we may have one cigarette and not acknowledge this to be a problem, so we have another. We are stuck in the pre-contemplation stage, perhaps allowing the arch enemy of "self-sabotage" to keep us there. We will need to progress around the stages of the cycle to get back in the right mindset, creating the resolve to break the habit again.

Being <u>aware</u> of this cycle can help us to regain control after a relapse more quickly, and even to bypass stages of the model, so that we can arrive back swiftly at action and maintenance.

 Exercise 28. Don't leave change to chance

46. How can I begin to break these habits long term?

It is true to say that we are creatures of habit. We lay down templates of behavior that we believe will help to meet our emotional needs. This process is usually unintentional and unconscious, and draws on past experiences and situations where something may have worked for us. However, it can lead us into patterns or habits which turn out to be problematic, as for example, when someone with a need for intimacy develops a habit of overeating as a means of providing a sense of internal "comfort."

Breaking these patterns requires that we understand how we "do" the pattern which leads us to the "point of no return"—the point at which we unconsciously reach for a cigarette or chocolate chip cookie, or start to bite our nails or grind our teeth. At this moment, we are in a **trance**

Ask yourself what emotional need or needs your habit is trying to address, using the list of emotional needs in Q.1. How can you meet these in more healthy or appropriate ways? What support will you need? Imagine how it will be to get your needs met in these better ways.

PRACTICAL TIP

Exercise 29. Move away from the point of no return

ON THE CD

state, completely and narrowly focused on the expectation of pleasure which we will experience once we take this final step. By understanding the thoughts, feelings, and actions that lead up to this point of no return and force us to act, we can bring the whole pattern into full consciousness. This enables us to make a choice to divert away from this critical point toward more resourceful behavior. The end result is that we feel better about ourselves and more in control.

47. What kind of attitude will help me keep focused on making positive changes?

The compassionate mind approach[33] to human psychology is gaining acceptance as a way of helping us to change unhealthy ways of thinking and behaving, particularly when the prospect of change can just seem too difficult. Developing a compassionate approach to our problems, for example, our relationship with food, alcohol or smoking, avoids the emotions of shame, blame, and self-criticism which in themselves can be overwhelming.

A compassionate approach has a number of elements:

Understanding what we're up against

For example, if we are struggling with obesity, we can understand how the food industry is geared to stoking our appetites, through including "eat more" chemicals in many foods and by promoting larger and larger portion sizes which are dense in fat, sugar, and calories. We can also understand that our human brains are designed to prompt us to eat when food is available, going back to times when our ancestors needed to forage and when food was often in short supply.

Taking control and responsibility for change

While the relationship with something like food is complex, understanding the problems we face can help us to move away from self-blaming and begin to help ourselves in a more compassionate and responsible way.

Being kind and supportive toward ourselves

Knowing that overeating is not entirely our fault, but that we *can* take responsibility for it, leads on to appreciating that we can gain control *over* it, too, if we can be kind and supportive to ourselves along the way. Kindness is not about treating ourselves to a big ice cream when we have managed to eat less for a week, but rather ensuring that we are meeting our real emotional needs, and this is a foundation stone to well-being (see Q.1).

We have already seen how important it is to switch off our **fight-or-flight response** (Chapter 2) and control our negative thinking (Chapter 3) in order to avoid intense emotions like anxiety, anger, and shame. However, there are areas of the brain, and particular hormones, which respond to self-compassion and to the kindness of others, and which can help to diffuse any sense of threat.

Compassion plays a key role in being able to develop happiness within ourselves and in our relationships with others, generating more resourceful thoughts, emotions, and actions which we can bring to bear on changing our habits. At the heart of developing compassion, is the desire to relieve our own and others' suffering. To develop compassionate motives, we need to understand our values and the kind of person we want to be.

PRACTICAL TIP Encourage yourself to take actions which are in your best interests, and the interests of others. Start with very small steps which are easy to do, and prepare yourself for practicing new skills you may need. Give yourself encouraging and kind thoughts along the way.

Exercise 30. Develop a compassionate mind

ON THE CD

So how can we develop a compassionate mind? Try the following activity which provides a significant first step.

CASE STUDY

William had tried giving up smoking four or five times since he turned thirty. He was now thirty-eight and really felt it was time to kick the habit once and for all. He realized that maybe this was the first time he was really <u>ready</u> to do it, noticing that when he ran through in his mind the last few times he had tried, he had quickly made up reasons to start again.

William began by thinking about those times he had started smoking again in order to come up with strategies he could employ if similar situations occurred. The last time was a break up of a relationship and he remembered his instant response was to phone a friend he knew who smoked and meet up with him. He devised a list of things he could do if/when he felt tempted to smoke, in order to avoid "the point of no return" (Exercise 29 on the CD-ROM), including, going out for a walk, watching his favorite comedy, going to his local cafe for a cup of tea, and to read the paper. He decided that for the next four weeks he would not meet smoking friends to give himself a chance to build his resolve before being in the face of temptation. He then tried the "compassionate self" visualization (Exercise 30 on the CD-ROM). He saw himself as more relaxed and calm, more open in his posture, leaning forward to hear and listen to people, not having to worry about smelling smoke.

After a very bad day at work, where his boss had ended up shouting at him, William went for a smoke with one of his old smoking buddies. Rather than berating himself and falling back into the habit, he went straight out for a run when we got home and practiced the visualization again, focusing on this as being an important part of the change process and something he could learn from. He also made a plan to practice a relaxation exercise at work whenever he felt stress building, rather than getting to the point he had that day.

Each non-smoking week that went by, William saved up his cigarette money and took his partner out for a meal or bought a new item of clothing as a reward. William felt that he now had a better understanding of his smoking behavior and had strategies in place to keep the "bully" of cigarettes at bay. He had one or two minor "slip-ups," but realizing that these were not significant, he then managed to stay off smoking long term.

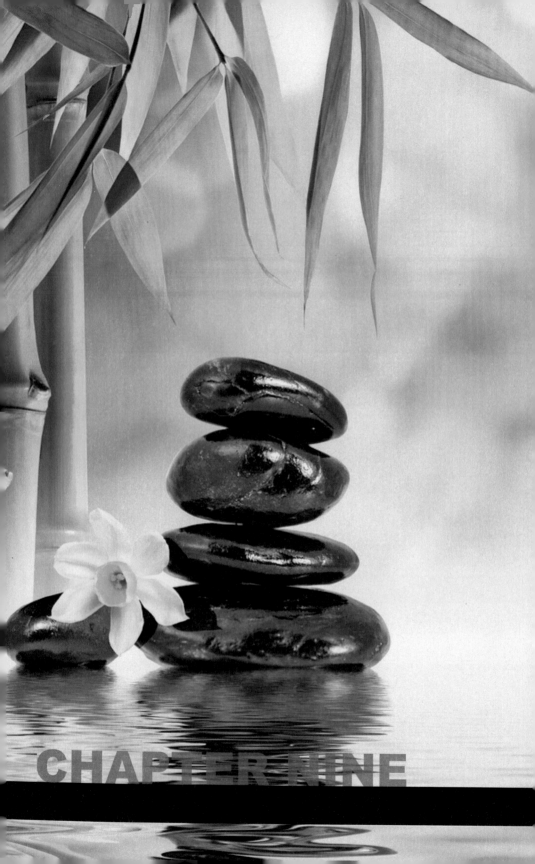

CHAPTER NINE

Toward Contentment

Martin Seligman's work over the past two decades has charted a new approach to living with "flexible optimism" and stimulated the growth of "positive psychology," which focuses on strengths rather than weaknesses. He shows how developing positive emotion in our lives can lead to better relationships, improved physical health, longer lives, and greater achievement.[34] In fact, one of the best predictors of successful aging is joy in living.[35]

Cultivating optimism and positive emotions leads to thinking about life's events in a more positive and hopeful light. Bad events are seen as being caused by external factors, specific to one area of life and likely to pass. The optimist is able to take comfort from their perceived strengths and other parts of their life where things are going well. When good events happen, they interpret them as a result of their own traits and abilities, that is, from more permanent causes than just good luck. Perceived success makes them try even harder, and they "get on a roll," feeling the benefits across all areas of their lives. This outlook contrasts with the pessimistic thinking associated with depression (Q.21). Staying hopeful is more than looking at the world through rose-tinted glasses. It is believing that they have both the will and the way that gives the optimist the resilience to cope with challenge and adversity.

Seligman argues that optimism can be learned. A key skill is learning to **reframe** your experiences in a more hopeful light. As we saw in Chapter 3 on negative thinking, an important factor in determining our happiness is not just what happens to us, but how we "frame" or give meaning to our experience. Learning to relax and engage the **observing self** gives us a chance to break out of disempowering ways of perceiving our reality—including our problems. We begin to see that there are alternative and more hopeful

We all know that feeling happy makes you smile, but did you know that putting a smile on your face makes you *feel* happier? James Laird and colleagues' research has shown that acting happy (or indeed, acting as if you are feeling any emotion), prompts us to feel that emotion.[36] So make your smile as wide as possible, lifting your eyebrow muscles upward and holding your happy expression for about twenty seconds.

ways of seeing our situation, which open up possibilities, rather than closing them down. It is like throwing open the shutters on a window and getting a wider, more inspiring view.

Positive emotions come from using our personal strengths, giving us a sense of gratification, and helping to make our lives more authentic. While eating a piece of cake may give us momentary pleasure, showing kindness by helping someone in need provides a longer lasting sense of gratification.

Strengths like kindness, courage, and integrity are enduring traits which can be built through teaching, practice, and persistence. Unlike talents, which we either have or do not have, we can choose to build our strengths and can feel elevated and inspired when we use them. Owning and choosing to use our strengths is at the heart of positive psychology. In contrast, many psychological interventions place individuals in a more passive role, by focusing on repairing the damage which might have been done to them via external events.

Exercise 31. Identify your signature strengths (and then use them)

ON THE CD

49. How does our view of the past influence well-being?

Our feelings about the past can range widely across emotions of contentment and fulfillment to bitterness, anger, and injustice. These emotions are determined by our thoughts about the past. Aaron T. Beck, an American psychiatrist who pioneered cognitive behavioral therapy (CBT) in the 1960s, demonstrated how thoughts influence feelings and behavior. Certainly, it is clear that the thoughts of depressed people are dominated by their negative interpretations of the past, and we have already looked at how learning to argue against these ways of thinking can be a way out of depression (see Chapter 3).

Our memories, thoughts and interpretations about the past can lock us into negative feelings which have a detrimental impact on our health and well-being. So how can we bring positive emotions about the past into our present? We can:

- Cultivate a sense of gratitude which helps us to savour and appreciate the good things that have happened in our lives.
- Forgive as a way of freeing ourselves from the power of past events and the intense negative emotions which may be attached to them.
- Focus on what went right for us in the past, including our successes, rather than what went wrong.
- Seek professional help to overcome post-traumatic stress (see Q.15).

Even though we cannot forget bad events, forgiving removes the emotional "sting" which blocks our capacity to experience contentment in the present. We often hold back from forgiving because of our sense of justice, as if forgiving takes away the right and proper need for revenge or for punishment of the transgressor. However, the only person we are punishing is *ourselves*, because our ongoing anger and bitterness diminishes our enjoyment of the present. Below is a five stage process for forgiving called REACH, developed by the psychologist, Everett Worthington and shown to have sizeable effects on reducing negative emotions and improving reported health:[37]

PRACTICAL TIP When you get into bed at night, spend a few moments remembering three reasons to be grateful for the day which has just ended.

R – recall the hurt in as objective a way as possible

E – empathize, or try to understand from the perpetrator's point of view why this person hurt you

A – give an altruistic gift of forgiveness, first recalling a time when you were forgiven

Some of these steps are challenging and it is important to seek professional support if you are experiencing intense emotion around particular memories.

C – commit yourself to forgive publicly, for example, by writing a letter to the perpetrator, writing it in a diary, or telling a trusted friend what you have done

Exercise 32. Focus on how far you have come

H – hold onto forgiveness by distracting away from the memories (Q.12(1)) and reminding yourself that you have forgiven

50. How do I increase my enjoyment of life (and experience peak performance)?

Have you ever become so absorbed in a pleasurable activity—reading, writing, gardening, painting, woodwork, sailing—only to realize later that two or more hours have passed in no time at all? It is not that your attention has wandered, but that you have been so focused, that time has disappeared and along with it, any sense of your surroundings. You will probably have felt positive, energized and totally aligned with the task at hand, freed from worry or anxiety. This is known as being in a state of **flow** and is a rewarding, even blissful, state which many performers, whether sports people, dancers, musicians, artists, or writers, utilize to make the difference between a competent and outstanding outcome.

The flow state, or being "in the zone" as athletes call it, has been defined and popularized by the world-famous psychologist, Mihály Csíkszentmihályi.[38] The necessary conditions for flow are that we are sufficiently challenged to test our skills, yet our skills are such that we can just meet the challenge. We are stretched to the limit and performing at our peak.

Csikszentmihalyi's work showed that in addition to having the necessary skills and techniques, peak performers are able to deliver consistently high levels of functioning on demand. This requires that they have an undivided focus of attention, a sense of control over what they are doing, with no emotions or worries about success or failure, and can lose the sense of self-consciousness which sometimes gets in the way of an excellent performance. It is almost as if their actions and awareness are merged, like a musician merging with her instrument. The activity becomes almost automatic and the involvement almost effortless. There is a feeling of total absorption, of being in the moment, without thinking about what needs to be done or what comes next.

 PRACTICAL TIP Flow occurs somewhere between the boredom of too little challenge and the anxiety of demands which are too much to handle. Identify activities where you experience a pleasurable level of challenge and absorption. Spend more time doing these and less time in low-challenge, apathy-inducing activities like watching TV.

How can we develop our capacity to get into "the zone," whether in our career, public performance, sport, or even just fully participating in a discussion or hobby? Here are some pointers:

- Check out your skill level. If you are still learning, you will need to stay more "conscious" of your actions and won't be ready to get into flow.

- Reduce performance anxiety with calming practices like **mindfulness**, meditation, or anchoring (see Q.6 and Q.9) which will lessen worrying and help you to re-evoke positive, past experiences.

- Trust the unconscious, rather than try to consciously focus on each movement or action. Thoughts and judgments will break the flow, as these activate the "analyzer" part of the brain, rather than the "integrator" part of the brain.

- Focus on the process and the moment, rather than on outcomes and external factors like how you look to others.

- Believe in the possibility of the impossible. Most people have no idea of what they are capable of doing and the limits are sky high!

Many performers mentally rehearse their peak performance repeatedly, which gives them a competitive edge. Researchers have shown that when you do this, the muscles you would normally be using show a tiny amount of stimulation.[39] In this way, the muscles "remember" the practice, in the same way that your brain remembers patterns of action and timing. You benefit from the mental rehearsal just as if you had practiced for real. Here is an activity for taking this on a step further, into peak performance.

Exercise 33. Access peak performance

ON THE CD

51. What can help me feel content and fulfilled?

One of our basic human needs is feeling a part of a wider community, a need to feel connected to something bigger than ourselves (see Q.1). Throughout this book we have explored the links between mental, emotional, and physical well-being. However, there is a fourth, spiritual dimension of well-being, which gives meaning to our existence and fulfills our need to connect to something beyond our egos— whether it is community, nature, a universal life force, or the Divine. Fostering our spirituality enables us to understand where we fit into the larger scheme of things. This can provide an important source of comfort and also a guide for our actions.

In an increasingly consumerist and individualistic society, it is easy to become focused on our own needs and wants.

Discovering our inner spirit and innermost values can enable us to move beyond the fear and negative thinking associated with our self-centeredness, to feeling more in touch with the welfare of other individuals, our communities and our environment. We are able to extend compassion, to give outward, and at the same time, experience a sense of wholeness within ourselves.

 PRACTICAL TIP Think of a time when you felt inspired, connected and fully "you." What personal values do you now see were in operation at the time?

Spirituality relates to our experience of being human, including the discovery of meaning and purpose in life and how we rise to the challenges life presents. It is about the connection we forge between that inner "spirit" and our outer world, but also the relationship we have with a "higher power" beyond and bigger than ourselves—whether that be "God," a universal consciousness, nature or some other source of inspiration. There is a growing body of evidence that cultivating a sense of spirituality or practicing a religion can have a positive impact on the way a patient perceives and experiences illness, and can be beneficial to both mental and physical health.[40] Religion can provide some people with an important faith community, with rituals and frameworks which can help them cope with life. However, we do not need to belong to an organized religion to feel that we have important personal values and a purpose in living.

Most religions and spiritual philosophies foster positive emotions like love and forgiveness, and Martin Seligman's work has demonstrated how happy people are more likely to demonstrate altruism.[41] Gratitude is another emotion linked to well-being. Research done by Robert Emmons and Michael McCullough showed that those who kept a daily gratitude journal—writing down things for which they were grateful on a daily basis—experienced higher levels of emotional <u>and</u> physical well-being.[42] Being grateful can transcend our own, narrow concerns and connect us to something positive outside ourselves, for example, the goodness of others, the beauty of nature, or the wonder of the divine. The experience of "transcendence" can be accompanied by a sense of awe, as when we appreciate a starry sky or a glorious sunset.

In 2008, the UK's Foresight Project published its findings from taking an independent and unparalleled look at how best to foster well-being within the nation. It considered the best available scientific evidence to identify the factors that influence an individual's mental development and well-being, from conception until death.[43] The project identified five suggestions for individual action in terms of promoting well-being, three of which are connected to the themes of this final piece and provide the final "Try this" activity:

Connect – With the people around you. With family, friends, colleagues, and neighbors. At home, work, school, or in your local community. Think of these as the cornerstones of your life and invest time in developing them. Building these connections will support and enrich you every day.

Give – Do something nice for a friend, or a stranger. Thank someone. Smile. Volunteer your time. Join a community group. Look out, as well as in. Seeing yourself, and your happiness, as linked to the wider community can be incredibly rewarding and creates connections with the people around you.

Take notice – Be curious. Catch sight of the beautiful. Remark on the unusual. Notice the changing seasons. Savour the moment, whether you are walking to work, eating lunch, or talking to friends. Be aware of the world around you and what you are feeling. Reflecting on your experiences will help you appreciate what matters to you.

Extracts from *Foresight Mental Capital and Wellbeing Project (2008). Final Project Report – Executive summary.* London: The Government Office for Science, p.22

Clayton was a fit seventy year old and had enjoyed a fulfilling work life as a team leader in a power plant. He had always felt part of a community and was chief organizer of social events, when his team would get together with other employees and bowl or enjoy quiz nights at the local bar. When he retired, he began to feel discontent. With his wife still working, he felt alone and unfulfilled during the day. He looked back at his life and felt bad about falling out with his brother many years before. He realized that he was still angry at his brother over a joint business venture which had gone wrong and had harbored ongoing resentment at the fact that his brother was better off than him. He knew he should forgive his brother and move on, but didn't know how. With his wife's support, they found a psychologist who was able to take him through a process of letting go of his anger and resentment, and forgiving his brother (Q.49). He began to understand why his brother had acted in the way he had, and decided to write him a letter of forgiveness, in which he recalled the good times they had shared together.

Clayton was reunited with his brother and they fondly remembered their boyhood fishing trips. They began to spend time fishing again, finding enjoyment in being alongside each other and appreciating the beauty of their surroundings. At these times, Clayton often experienced a strong feeling of being at one with his brother and with everything around him. He had never been a religious man, but was comforted and uplifted by these moments, and began to take up a regular practice of spending contemplative time at home.

Clayton's brother introduced Clayton to friends who regularly met and organized charity events. He discovered that helping other people gave him real pleasure and a sense of belonging to a community again. Quickly his retirement became a chance to do things he had always wanted to do, as well as things he hadn't even thought about before, and he felt blessed to have the time to discover new ways of feeling fulfilled.

Appendix

The CD-ROM contains a selection of activities, links, four audio recordings for relaxation, and printable exercises to put the information and ideas from the book into practice.

Audio Recordings

Track 1: 7/11 breathing and body scan

- *Two breathing and body relaxation exercises for fast stress reduction.*

Track 2: Mindfulness breathing

- *An exercise in mindfulness-based stress reduction that focuses on the breath.*

Track 3: Step down

- *A visualization for relaxation, based on hypnotherapy.*

Track 4: An anchor for calm

- *A relaxing exercise to create a mental anchor for calm, based on neuro-linguistic programming (NLP)*

References

CHAPTER 1

1   Griffin, J. and Tyrrell, I. Human Givens—A new approach to emotional health and clear thinking, pp. 93-133. Chalvington, UK: HG Publishing.

2   Kabat-Zinn, J. (2004) *Full Catastrophe Living. How to cope with stress, pain and illness using mindfulness meditation.* London: Piatkus.

3   Ludwig, D. and Kabat-Zinn, J (2008) "Mindfulness in Medicine." *Journal of the American Medical Association* 300 (11) 1350-1352.

4   Walker Atkinson, W. (1908) *Thought Vibration or the Law of Attraction in the Thought World* Chicago: The New Thought Publishing Company. Re-edited and republished in 2008 by Seed of Life Publishing, USA.

CHAPTER 2

5   Kerkhof, A. (2010) *Stop Worrying* (p.24). Maidenhead: Open University Press (McGraw-Hill)

6   Gournay, K. (2010) *Coping with Phobias and Panic* (p.4). London: Sheldon Press

7   Wolpe, J. (1969) *The Practice of Behavior Therapy*. Oxford. Pergamon Press.

8   Griffin, J. and Tyrell I. (2005) "PTSD: why some techniques for treating it work so fast." *Human Givens Journal*, 12, (3).

9   Gournay, K. (2010) *Coping with Phobias and Panic* (p.24). London: Sheldon Press.

10 Shapiro, F. (2001) *EMDR: Eye Movement Desensitization of Reprocessing: Basic Principles, Protocols and Procedures* (2nd edition). New York: Guilford Press.

CHAPTER 3

11 Deikman, A. (1982) *The Observing Self: Mysticism and Psychotherapy*. Boston: Beacon Press.

12 Peterson, C., Maier, S. and Seligman, M. (1995).*Learned Helplessness: A Theory for the Age of Personal Control*. New York: Oxford University Press.

13 Griffin, J. (1997) "The Origin of Dreams." *The Therapist Ltd.* Chalvington, UK: HG Publishing.

14 DeRubeis, R. et al. (2008) "Cognitive therapy versus medication for depression: treatment outcomes and neural mechanisms." *Nature Reviews Neuroscience,* 9, 788-796.

15 Teasdale, J. Segal, Z. Williams, et al. (2000) "Prevention of relapse/recurrence in major depression by mindfulness-based cognitive therapy." *Journal of Consulting and Clinical Psychology,* 68, 615-623.

16 Ma, S. and Teasdale, J. (2004) "Mindfulness-based cognitive therapy for depression: Replication and exploration of differential relapse prevention effects." *Journal of Consulting and Clinical Psychology,* 72, 31-40.

17 http://ww.hgfoundation.com/documents/Luton_Study_BPS.pdf, (last accessed March 2013).

CHAPTER 4

18 Siegel, D. (2012) *The Developing Mind: How relationships and the brain interact to shape who we are* (2nd edition). New York: Guilford Press.

CHAPTER 5

19 Ader, R. et al. (1995) Psychoneruoimmunology: interactions between the nervous system and immune system. *Lancet* 345 (99).

20 Martin, P. (2005) *The Sickening Mind: Brain, behavior, immunity and disease* (p54). London: Harper Perennial.

21 http://www.ibshypnosis.com/IBSresearch.html, (last accessed Nov 2012).

22 O'Hanlon, W. and Hexum, A. (1991) *An Uncommon Casebook: The complete clinical work of Milton H Erickson, MD.* London: WW Norton.

23 Melzack, R. and Wall, P. (1965) "Pain mechanisms: a new theory." *Science,* 150, 971-9.

24 Martin, P. (2005) *The Sickening Mind: Brain, behavior, immunity and disease* (p. 250). London: Harper Perennial.

CHAPTER 6

25   Griffin, J. (2005) *Freedom from Addiction: The secret behind successful addiction busting.* Chalvington, UK: HG Publishing.

CHAPTER 7

26   www.attitudespecialist.co.nz/self-esteem.html, (last accessed Nov 2012).

27   Lovelace, R. (1990) *Stress Master.* Chichester, UK: John Wiley & Sons.

28   Wiseman, R. (2012) *Rip It Up. The radically new approach to changing your life.* London: Macmillan.

29   University of Notre Dame (2001) *Mr Nice Guy: Being genetically disagreeable gets you paid at work.* Mendoza College of Business. Available at www.medicalnewstoday.com/articles/232830.php.

30   Borg, J. (2010) *Body Language: 7 Easy Lessons to Master the Silent Language.* FT Press.

CHAPTER 8

31   Prochaska, J. and DiClemente, C. (1984) *The Transtheoretical Approach: Toward a Systematic Eclectic Framework.* Homewood, IL, USA: Dow Jones Irwin.

32   Worrall, P., and Cooper, C. (2012) *The Quality of Working Life. Managers' Wellbeing, Motivation and Productivity.* Available at http://www.mbsportal.bl.uk/taster/subjareas/mgmt/cmi/134042qualitywl12.pdf.

33   Gilbert, P. (2009) *The Compassionate Mind.* London: Constable Robinson.

CHAPTER 9

34   Seligman, M. (2003) *Authentic Happiness.* London: Nicholas Brealey.

35   Vaillant, G. (2000) "Adaptive mental mechanisms: their role in Positive Psychology." *American Psychologist* 55 89-98.

36   Flack Jr., W. Laird, J. Cavallaro, L.(1974) "Separate and combined effects of facial expressions and bodily postures on emotional feelings." *Journal of Personality and Social Psychology* 29 (4) 475-486.

37 Worthington, E. (Ed) (1998) *Dimensions of Forgiveness: Psychological research and theological perspectives.* Philadelphia: Templeton Foundation Press.

38 Csikszentmilalyi, M. (1992) *Flow: The Psychology of Happiness.* London: Riderche.

39 Jacobson, E. (1932) "Electrophysiology of mental activities." *American Journal of Psychology* 44a.

40 Bauer-Wu, S. and Farran, C. (2005) "Meaning in life and psycho-spiritual functioning: a comparison of breast cancer survivors and healthy women." *Journal of Holistic Nursing* 23 172-190.

41 Diener, E. and Seligman, M. (2002) Very Happy People. *Psychological Science* 13 81-84.

42 Emmons, R. and McCullough, M. (2004) *The Psychology of Gratitude.* Oxford: Oxford University Press.

43 *Foresight Mental Capital and Wellbeing Project* (2008) London: The Government Office for Science.

Glossary

Amygdala

The amygdala is an almond shaped structure deep within the limbic brain, which is involved in the processing of emotions such as fear, anger and pleasure, and determining what memories are stored and where the memories are stored in the brain. This appears to depend on how huge an emotional response an event invokes. In the case of high emotional arousal (perceived danger), the amygdala triggers the fight-or-flight response via the hypothalamus.

Adrenaline

Adrenaline is a hormone produced by the adrenal glands during high stress or exciting situations. This powerful hormone is part of the human body's acute stress response system, also called the "fight-or-flight" response. It works by stimulating the heart rate, contracting blood vessels, and dilating air passages, all of which work to increase blood flow to the muscles and oxygen to the lungs, preparing the body for "action."

Cognitive Behavioral Therapy

Cognitive behavioral therapy (CBT) was pioneered by Dr Aaron Beck. It is a form of psychological therapy which examines the relationship between thoughts (cognitions) and how they influence feelings and behaviors. CBT interventions are designed to help people identify negative patterns of behavior and to develop and practice more positive and healthy ways of thinking. It is used to treat depression, anxiety, anger, chronic pain, and other conditions with a significant psychological component.

Dopamine

Dopamine is a neurotransmitter that helps control the brain's reward and pleasure centers, as well as helping to regulate movement and emotional responses. It enables us not only to see rewards, but to take action to move toward them.

Fight-or-flight Response

Originally discovered by the great Harvard physiologist Walter Cannon, this response is hard-wired into our brains to enable our physical survival in times of danger. The response corresponds to an area in the base of the brain called the hypothalamus, which, when stimulated by the amygdala, initiates a sequence of nerve cell firing and chemical release (including, noradrenaline and cortisol) that prepares our body for running or fighting. In this survival mode, along with a series of physiological changes that occur, the rational mind is suppressed, and we are unable to think strategically, nor cultivate positive attitudes or beliefs.

Flow

Flow is the mental state in which a person in an activity is fully immersed in a feeling of energized focus, full involvement, and success in the process of the activity. Proposed by Mihály Csíkszentmihályi, the positive psychology concept has been applied within a variety of fields. In flow, the emotions are not just contained and channeled, but positive, energized, and aligned with the task at hand. In a state of depression or anxiety, we are barred from flow. The hallmark of flow is a feeling of spontaneous joy, even rapture, while performing a task, although flow can also be described as a deep focus on nothing but the activity—not even oneself or one's emotions.

Human Givens

The Human Givens approach is an organizing idea, drawn from both ancient wisdom and the latest scientific understandings from neurobiology and psychology, which provides a holistic, scientific framework for understanding the way that individuals and society work. At its core is the highly empowering idea that human beings, like all organic beings, come into this world with a set of needs. If those needs are met appropriately, it is not possible to suffer from mental ill-health, including depression, psychosis, and addictive or self-harming behavior.

Hypnotherapy

Hypnotherapy utilizes hypnosis as a way of helping people to change unwanted patterns of behavior. Leading exponent of hypnosis, psychiatrist Milton H. Erickson, clearly demonstrated the clinical value of this tool, which accesses the state of consciousness in which nature programs the brain and can reprogram it. The Ericksonian approach departed from traditional hypnosis by stressing the importance of interaction with the patient and actively engaging with their inner resources and experiential life (in contrast to issuing standardized instructions to a passive subject). In doing so, it revolutionized the practice of hypnotherapy and brought many original concepts of communication and therapeutic working into the field.

Limbic system

Sometimes known as the "emotional brain," the limbic system is the set of brain structures that forms the inner border of the cortex and is considered to include the amygdala, which signals stimuli involving reward or fear to the cortex, and the hippocampus, which is required for the formation of long-term memories.

Metaphor

An idea which is used to suggest a likeness or analogy between one thing and another. We all use metaphors to describe our situation or condition. Used therapeutically, a metaphor such as a word, phrase or story might be offered to the client to give them a different way of seeing their problem.

Mindfulness

A technique for turning off busy thoughts, derived from Buddhist meditation practices, it involves focusing awareness on moment-by-moment experience, for example, focusing on the breath entering and leaving the nose.

Mindfulness-based Stress Reduction (MBSR)

A structured group program that employs mindfulness meditation to alleviate suffering associated with physical, psychosomatic and psychiatric disorders. The program is non-religious and is based upon a systematic procedure to develop enhanced awareness of moment-to-moment experience of perceptible mental processes. It has been shown to be effective in alleviating chronic pain, depression, and anxiety disorders.

Neocortex

The neocortex is the more recently evolved part of the brain in humans and mammals. Responsible for complex mental activity, it almost completely covers the rest of the brain and comprises four major lobes.

Neuro-Linguistic Programing

Neuro-Linguistic Programing, or NLP, was first developed by Richard Bandler and John Grinder in the 1970s and is now widely applied within psychotherapy, interpersonal communications and management training. Through understanding how we structure and give meaning to our internal, subjective world, NLP enables us to learn how to choose our emotional state, rather than being prey to unhelpful emotions, especially at times when we want to stay resourceful.

Observing self

A natural mechanism human beings have to step outside of our thoughts, feelings, and actions and look in on ourselves, so that the world can be seen more objectively. It is a fundamental state of awareness which can be used by therapists to help a client identify the patterns of conditioning which need to change. The term was coined by the psychiatrist, Dr Arthur Deikman.

Nocebo

Nocebo means "I will harm." The nocebo effect is the experience of negative health outcomes following a treatment that should have no effect.

Placebo

The literal meaning of placebo is "I shall please." The placebo effect has been much researched and refers to health benefits produced by treatments without demonstrable substance, and that should have no effect.

Psychoneuroimmunology

Following the discovery in 1974 by Robert Ader, a psychologist, that the immune system, like the brain, can learn, psychoneuroimmunology has become a leading-edge medical science, exploring the links between the mind and emotions, nervous system, hormone system, and immune system.

Reframing

A core skill employed in counseling and psychotherapy, reframing addresses how a person "frames" their experience. It is used to replace a negative, narrow, inaccurate, or unhelpful way of interpreting their experience with a more hopeful, richer one that opens up new possibilities.

Useful Resources

1. **Laying the Foundations of Emotional Health and Well-being**
   Relax CD with Piers Bishop by HG publishing, available at: http://www. humangivens.com/publications/relax.html.

   Dyer, W. (2004) *The Power Of Intention. Change the way you look at things and the things you look at will change.* Carlsbad, Ca: Hay House Inc.

2. **Dealing with Stress, Anxiety, Panic, and Worry**
   Griffin, J. and Tyrrell, I. (2007) *How to Master Anxiety.* Chalvington, UK: HG Publishing.

   Bourne, E. (2000) *The Anxiety & Phobia Workbook* (3rd edition). Oakland, CA: New Harbinger Publications Inc.

3. **Controlling Negative Thinking and Avoiding Depression**
   Williams, M., Teasdale, J,, Sega,l Z. and Kabat-Zinn, J. (2007) *The Mindful Way Through Depression.* New York: Guilford Press.

   www.clinical-depression.co.uk

   Depression quiz, recovery programme and learning path available for people suffering from depression, those living with them, and therapists treating them.

4. **Reducing Anger**
   Dawes, M. and Winn, D. (1999) *Managing The Monkey: How to diffuse the conflicts that can lead to violence in the workplace.* Chalvington, UK: HG Publishing.

   Griffin, J., and Tyrrell, I. (2008) *Release from Anger. Practical help for controlling unreasonable rage.* UK:H.G Publishing.

5. **Improving Physical Health and Sleep**
   Cole, F. et al. (2005) *Overcoming chronic pain: A self-help guide using cognitive behavioural techniques.* London: Constable & Robinson.

   Espie, C. (2006) *Overcoming insomnia and sleep problems: A self-help guide using cognitive behavioural techniques.* London: Constable & Robinson Ltd.

   Kabat-Zinn, J. (2004) *Full Catastrophe Living. How to cope with stress, pain and illness using mindfulness meditation.* London: Piatkus.

   Mental Health Foundation (2011) *Sleep Well: Your Pocket Guide To Better Sleep.* London: Mental Health Foundation (free).

6. **Setting Goals and Boosting Motivation**
   Hadfield, S. (2012) *Brilliant Positive Thinking: Transform your outlook and face the future with confidence and optimism.* Harlow: Pearson Education Ltd.

7. **Enhancing Assertiveness, Self-esteem and Confidence**
   Robinson, D. (1997) *Too nice for your own good: How to stop making 9 self-sabotaging mistakes.* New York: Warner Books Inc.

   Fennell, M. (2009) *Overcoming Low Self Esteem: A self help guide using Cognitive Behavioral Techniques.* London: Constable and Robinson Ltd.

9. **Changing Unhelpful Habits and Patterns**
   Goss, K. (2011) *The Compassionate Mind Approach to Beating Overeating. Using compassion focused therapy.* London: Constable.

   Griffin, J. (2005) *Freedom from Addiction: The secret behind successful addiction busting.* Chalvington, UK: HG Publishing.

Prochaska, J., Norcross, J. and DiClemente, C. (1994) *Changing For Good: The revolutionary program that explains the six stages of change and teaches you how to free yourself from bad habits.* New York: W. Morrow.

10. **Toward Contentment**

Buzan, T. (1988) *Make the Most of Your Mind.* London: Pan Books.

Seligman, M. (2003) *Authentic Happiness.* London: Nicholas Brealey Publishing.

Authentic Happiness http://www.authentichappiness.sas.upenn.edu/register.aspx

Develop insights into yourself and the world around you through these scientifically tested questionnaires, surveys and scales.

Valliant, G. (2002) Aging Well. New York: Little, Brown

General

Cognitive Behavioural Therapy

Beck Institute for Cognitive Behavioral Therapy http://www.beckinstitute.org.

An international training and resource center for health and mental health professionals, educators, and students worldwide.

Carlson, R. (1997) *Stop Thinking and Start Living: Common-sense strategies for discovering lifelong happiness.* London: Element.

The MoodGYM http://moodgym.anu.edu.au.

A free self-help program to teach cognitive behavioral therapy skills to people vulnerable to depression and anxiety.

Powell, T. (2009) *The Mental Health Handbook. A cognitive behavioural approach.* Milton Keynes: Speechmark Publishing.

Compassionate Mind approach

Gilbert, P. (2009) *The Compassionate Mind.* London: Constable Robinson.

Compassionate Mind Foundation www.compassionatemind.co.uk.

Human Givens approach

Griffin, J. and Tyrrell, I. (2004) *Human Givens. A new approach to emotional health and clear thinking.* Chalvington, UK: HG Publishing.

Hypnotherapy

Alman, B. and Lambrou, P. (1992) *Self-Hypnosis. The complete manual for health and self-change* (2nd edition). New York: Brunner/Mazel.

Erickson, M. H. and Rossi, E. L. (1979) *Hypnotherapy: An Exploratory Casebook.* New York: Irvington.

Mindfulness

Kabat-Zinn, J. (2005) *Coming to our Senses: Healing ourselves and the world through mindfulness.* New York: Piatkus.

Siegel, D. (2007) *The Mindful Brain: Reflection and attunement in the cultivation of well-being.* London: WW Norton.

Neuro-Linguistic Programing

Bandler, R. and Grinder, J. (1979) *Frogs into Princes: Neuro Linguistic Programing.* Moab, UT: Real People Press.

O'Connor, J. (2001) *NLP Workbook. A practical guide to achieving the results you want.* London: Element.

Positive Psychology

Boniwell, I. (2008) *Positive Psychology in a Nutshell* (2nd edition) London: Personal Well-being Centre.

Index

NLP. *See* neuro-linguistic
   programming
nocebo effect, 62
non-verbal communication,
   78–79

O
observing self, 35, 52, 93
obsessive-compulsive disorder
   (OCD), 29–30
OCD. *See* obsessive-compulsive
   disorder
optimism, 93–94

P
panic attacks
   definition, 20
   factors, 20–21
   physical symptoms, 21
past feelings, influence,
   94–96
perfectionism, 41
phobia
   definition, 24
   psychological treatment
      cognitive behavioral
         therapy, 25–26
      systematic desensitization,
         25
      visual/kinesthetic
         dissociation, 26
physical health
   affecting ways, 56–57
   mind power, 58–59
placebo effect, 61
PNI. *See*
   psychoneuroimmunology
positive emotions, 93–94
positive psychology,
   93–94
positive visualization, 9

post-traumatic stress disorder
   (PTSD)
   occurrence, 27
   psychological treatments, 28
      eye movement
         desensitization and
         reprocessing, 29
      visual/kinesthetic
         dissociation, 28
pre-contemplation, 86
programing state, 9
psychoneuroimmunology
   (PNI), 56
PTSD. *See* post-traumatic
   stress disorder

R
rapid eye movement (REM),
   9, 29
REACH, forgiving process,
   95–96
real worries, 18
reframe, 44, 59, 93
relapse, 85, 87
relaxation response
   characteristics, 7
   description, 5
   techniques
      breathing and body scan, 8
      mindfulness meditation,
         8–9
      visualization, 9–10
REM. *See* rapid eye movement
resource anchoring,
   17–18
reticular formation, 11
rewind technique
   in phobia, 26
   in post-traumatic stress
      disorder, 28
rumination, 18, 39